'*Searching for a Rose Garden* is an e
in which contributors reflect on the ...., setbacks, and ongoing
challenges in contesting and supplanting psychiatry. There is an arresting
quality to these essays, which express the urgency of needing to find other
ways of caring, and are grounded in a deep appreciation of other ways
of being. The transformative effects of the collective knowledge woven
together in this book will reverberate for decades to come.'

Dr Richard Ingram, Independent Mad Studies Researcher

'A vital contribution to the building of Mad Studies as a discipline grounded
in activist scholarship. This is a comprehensive and accessible must-read
for those interested in building real alternatives to the limited, and often
damaging, approaches to madness and distress that dominate today. Its
scope is impressive, drawing together a wide range of contributions to
show the best of survivor knowledge and practice, whilst raising questions
concerning the politics of inclusion, identities and co-production within
this field. It serves as a record and celebration of, and a challenge to,
survivor knowledge and activism; in doing so it preserves and provokes
in equal measure.'

Dr Brigit McWade, Sociology Department, Lancaster University

'A profoundly important volume and a herculean effort. Comprehensive,
modern, bold, accessible, survivor-produced research, knowledge and
practice. *Searching for a Rose Garden* offers concrete examples of people
rejecting and altering "mental health" systems around the world. This is a
must-read for anyone who has ever heard the word "psychiatry".'

Lauren J Tenney, PhD, MPhil, MPA, Psychiatric Survivor

SEARCHING FOR A ROSE GARDEN

CHALLENGING PSYCHIATRY, FOSTERING MAD STUDIES

Edited by
Jasna Russo and Angela Sweeney

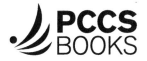

First published 2016

PCCS Books Ltd
Wyastone Business Park
Wyastone Leys
Monmouth
NP25 3SR
contact@pccs-books.co.uk
www.pccs-books.co.uk

British Library Cataloguing in Publication data: a catalogue record
for this book is available from the British Library.

ISBN 978-1-910919-23-1

Cover design by Phipps Design
Typeset in the UK by Raven Books
Typeset using Minion Pro and Myriad Pro
Cover image and image editing by Tünya Özdemir – www.tektek.de
Printed by Lightning Source

CONTENTS

SURVIVOR-CONTROLLED PRACTICE

WORKING IN PARTNERSHIP

THE SEARCH GOES ON

Foreword

Brenda A LeFrançois

Mad Studies is not about separatism, empire building or marginalisation; nor is it about academic or professional elitism. Instead, Mad Studies centres the knowledges of those deemed mad, bolstered on the periphery by the important relationships, work and support of allies – or by those who comport themselves as mad-positive. This allows those of us deemed mad to formulate and advance our own understandings, theories, research, actions, practices and knowledges, each of which carries an inherently enhanced credibility *because* of direct experience. We might refer to this as mad activist scholarship, a form of knowledge production or collective intellectual contribution that is embedded in Mad community interventions and actions. At the same time, this form of knowledge production and activism also acknowledges not needing to resist and toil wholly on our own to dismantle what has become an all too economically powerful and deeply politically entrenched psychiatric system. The Mad Studies project offers us a way forward in revealing or creating knowledges that do not contain the distortions and harmfulness proffered by a biomedical psychiatry that is so distant from our lived realities. Also, it allows for the choice to integrate any useful existing or newly developing knowledges, actions and interventions proffered by critical academics, radical professionals and other allies.

Mad Studies, however, takes place within and without academia, but never without community. Richard Ingram, in coining the term Mad Studies in 2008, conceptualised it as an 'in/discipline' (Ingram, 2015; 2016). He explains that in some spaces like academia 'sly normality' (Mills, 2014; 2013) must be performed, while at the same time in mad community spaces the queerness of thoughts and behaviours – or the indiscipline that may characterise them – is known, honoured and lived (Ingram, 2016), incomprehensible as that may be to the sanestream. Examples of where Mad Studies as an in/discipline is occurring in our various local communities include the reading group in the Netherlands initiated by Grietje Keller (Keller, 2015), the North East Mad Studies Forum[1] in England, and the group in Moncton, Canada initiated by Rachel LeBlanc, to name just a few. There are also the well-known courses in academia in Canada, Scotland and England. This book offers us several other examples of Mad Studies – of 'thinking environments' – ranging from survivor-produced knowledges to survivor-created and survivor-controlled practices to partnerships in research and higher education teaching, some lesser known, with little having been written about them previously.

In my view, this extraordinary volume represents a crucial and unprecedented account of what Mad Studies is all about. Notably, it is almost wholly written by psychiatric survivors, with the exception of only three chapters co-authored in partnership with allies, in addition to the last chapter written solely by ally Reima Maglajlic. I first met Reima in England in the mid-1990s, and it seems not accidental that I encounter her here again, decades later, in this book. We both studied under the late Professor David Brandon – in Rea's words, 'one of the first mental-health-system-survivors-cum-professors-of-social-work' (p210). He was a formidable and leading figure in the psychiatric survivor community in the UK from around the 1970s until his untimely death in 2001, and the education we received from him was equally formidable. Initially through that mad activist education under David's guidance and tutelage, and later through engaging in community actions and independent reading, I became familiar with and learned much from the previous writings and activism of most of the contributors of this volume. In fact, I have been profoundly influenced at different times over the past 20 years by the writings, activism and courage of so many of them.

And now, finally, we have this book, which I envisage will be taken up as foundational in Mad Studies. Many of the thoughts and teachings contained within it are authored by people who have been working in the trenches for a long time to create mad spaces in practice, education and research. In effect, we have a book in our hands that we can now dip in and out of, and which might just be able to sustain us in those bleak moments when the work we all do seems too overwhelming, dangerous or unachievable. Filled with poignant analyses, strong political commitments and a passion for social justice, the chapters weave together a multitude of ideas, perspectives and experiences. In reading it, sometimes I could feel the words resonating in my bones; sometimes I

---

1. See http://madstudiesne.weebly.com/

found myself cheering as the words on the page dared to say out loud what others will not – the simple yet complex truths that others do not have the courage or honesty to speak.

As such, this volume contains so many of the important arguments – mad activist arguments – that link together the diverse issues subsumed within the umbrella of Mad Studies. It offers critiques of biomedical psychiatry, allowing us to appreciate anew why different and mad-informed ways of understanding and addressing distress and extreme states of mind are of such central importance. In addition, it tackles head-on issues of psychiatric survivor exclusions linked to assumptions about (il)legitimacy and (lack of) credibility, both within and outside of psychiatry. As well, it interrogates the fairly consistent appropriation and distorting of psychiatric survivor contributions over time and across space.

Both the breadth and depth of this book's focus and discussion were at times arresting for me to read; I am left thinking through issues that are pressing but have perhaps not been invoked or developed in writing before. Here, we find warnings of what might happen when partnerships harm more than help, or when our goals lose their initially unabashed political grounding, or when we become corrupted by a hierarchical and competitive academic culture that is detached from the mad community and people's everyday lives. Here, we learn about the problems that arise when mad identity remains undisclosed, as well as analyses of the fragility and the impossibility of mad identity. Here, too, we are asked to think about and confront racism within and outside of psychiatry, including systemic whiteness not just within psy-systems but also within the mad movement itself, the privileging of white survivor contributions and the erasure of cultural memory when it is not consistent with established white Western understandings.

All this and so much more within its pages make this volume both vital to our movement and perhaps of fundamental importance to the evolution of Mad Studies. In short, this book has provided a locus for exposing – and being recognised for – the kind of meaningful meaning-(un)making that is possible within Mad Studies.

Brenda A LeFrançois

References

Keller G (2015). *Theory as Healing: Mad Studies reading groups in Amsterdam.* Conference presentation. Making Sense of Mad Studies conference, 30 September 2015; Durham University, UK.

Ingram R (in press). Doing Mad Studies: making (non)sense together. *Intersectionalities* 5(2).

Ingram R (2015). *Doing Mad Studies: the subject and object at a boiling point.* Conference presentation. Making Sense of Mad Studies conference, 1 October 2015; Durham University, UK.

Mills C (2014). Sly normality: between quiescence and revolt. In: Burstow B, LeFrançois BA, Diamond S (eds). *Psychiatry Disrupted: theorizing resistance and crafting the (r)evolution.* Montréal: McGill/Queen's University Press (pp194–207).

Mills C (2013). *Decolonizing Global Mental Health: the psychiatrization of the majority world.* London: Routledge.

Introduction

Jasna Russo and Angela Sweeney

This book emerged from the international conference 'Searching for a Rose Garden: fostering real alternatives to psychiatry', held in Berlin in September 2011. Organised by the Association for Protection against Psychiatric Violence, this unique two-day event aimed to introduce and explore alternatives to psychiatry that build on survivors' own knowledges and understandings of madness and distress. The conference was announced as 'bringing together world leaders in the field' and providing 'an important chance to reflect in depth on these innovative approaches: their origins and potential, the prerequisites for their development and the difficulties they face'.[1]

The event attracted around 220 people from 10 European countries, the US and Australia. Many more could not be there because of the limited size of the venue and the lack of travel bursaries. The enthusiasm with which the conference programme was immediately and widely received confirmed that there is a serious dearth of gatherings of this kind globally. This, as well as the unique atmosphere of the conference, gave us the impetus to begin conceptualising this book. People with 'lived experience' are increasingly invited as speakers to mental health, social work and psychiatric conferences. But we rarely constitute the majority of key speakers, we rarely come from several different countries, and frequently our contributions are reduced to personal recovery stories. What made this conference unique was that, building on their experiential knowledge, speakers presented their research, theoretical, conceptual and practice work. Placing this expertise centre-stage made it an intense and unusual experience, as this feedback from one participant from Belgium demonstrates:

---

1. The conference programme and report (in German) are available at http://www.weglaufhaus.de/kongress/

I felt that I'm not a professional who visits the place where (ex) psychiatric patients will present their views, and then I can decide if I believe them, but I felt that I'm visiting a place where the real knowledge of this field lies.[2]

We were both involved in this conference – Jasna as the main organiser and Angela as a delegate and speaker – and are still indelibly affected by its galvanising atmosphere. Our hope is to open up another such space through this collection. To achieve this we have widened the original group of conference speakers and sought further authors whose work offers a distinctive contribution to the field. Our search for contributions focused on what we consider to be true alternatives to the biomedical model, both in research and practice.

Initially we kept the conference title as the working title for the book. However, the subsequent contributions we received ultimately led us out of the 'field' of psychiatry and alternatives to psychiatry and we found ourselves at home in Mad Studies. This term was not known in Europe back in 2011 when the conference was held, or at least not to our knowledge. As described by the editors of the first book to introduce Mad Studies, it is 'a project of inquiry, knowledge production, and political action devoted to the critique and transcendence of psy-centred ways of thinking, behaving, relating, and being' (LeFrançois et al, 2013: 13). For us, Mad Studies offers a new and powerful framework that connects the authors' voices and situates their groundbreaking work.

The authors have their own views on the capitalisation of the word 'mad'. We have on principle respected their preferences, which explains the variance in the chapters. However we have chosen to capitalise the term 'Mad Studies' to denote its status as a distinct field of scholarship and to convey the politicisation that we feel is inherent to the endeavour.

The contributions are presented in four sections. The first section sets the scene for the book, reminding us why radically different approaches to madness and distress are needed (chapters by Mary O'Hagan, Bhargavi Davar and Beth Filson). We also discuss the potential contribution of those whose knowledges have traditionally been excluded from the field (chapter by Peter Beresford) and highlight at the very beginning the pitfalls and dangers of joining a field dominated by biomedical approaches to human crises (the chapter by Darby Penney and Laura Prescott).

The next two sections, 'Survivor-Produced Knowledge' and 'Survivor-Controlled Practice', feature examples of our contributions to theory and research

---

2. E-mail received on 6 September 2011.

on one hand and to practice on the other. Inevitably, the contents of these sections overlap as theory and practice are inseparable. The section on theory and research aims to provide an insight into academic work that is being undertaken autonomously, not in collaboration with clinical academics, and that signifies a radical departure from the dominant paradigm. Besides our own contributions focusing on survivors in research and theory building, this section includes Colin King's chapter on whiteness in psychiatry and its consequences, Clare Shaw's re-conceptualisation of self-harm and David Webb's call for a radical re-thinking of suicidality. This section ends with Erick Fabris's reflections on how we can stop investing in models that will only be turned into the opposite of what they were intended to be.

The section on practice includes authors' descriptions and discussions of the concrete support work they are developing or providing. When compiling the conference programme, it proved hard to find existing services that were conceptualised and led by survivors. The organising group deliberately decided to leave aside well-established alternatives to mainstream psychiatric provision, such as Soteria, Windhorse or Open Dialogue, which all have one known professional (non-survivor) figure behind them. Instead, we focused on lesser-known projects that grew from collective first-person knowledge of people on the receiving end of mainstream services. It is hard to find projects that fulfill this criteria and are still operating; over time, projects started by survivors tend to lose their initial distinctive characteristics and become taken over by professional workers until they turn into just another community psychiatric service.

This has happened, for instance, to the Berlin Runaway House, whose provider, the Association for Protection Against Psychiatric Violence, organised the 'Searching for a Rose Garden' conference. Besides several fundamental changes that have occurred to this survivor-founded residential service in the course of its 20-year existence, one of the core rules that at least half of the service's workers have to have personal psychiatric experience was officially abolished in March 2014. Unfortunately we were unable to obtain an account that captured these significant developments in all their complexity, but we hope the time will come when there will be a comprehensive analysis of all that occurred that will provide the case study that this global phenomenon deserves.

Alongside chapters showing the immense transformative potential of survivor-defined forms of support (those by Shery Mead and Beth Filson, Patsy Staddon, Maths Jesperson and Zofia Rubinsztajn), other contributions in this section also describe a struggle for recognition and resources (chapters by Renuka Bhakta, Terry Simpson and, again, Patsy Staddon), as well as some of the side effects of such struggles that can ultimately lead services down the path of 'professionalisation', compromising their core values and principles (the chapter by Zofia Rubinsztajn).

We decided to devote the last section to 'Working in Partnership' because this remains the most common way in which service users and survivors contribute to research and practice. We appreciate the openness and honesty with which authors have written about their joint work (chapter by Dolly Sen and Anna Sexton), and are proud to feature reflections from the partnership that pioneered peer work within the psychiatric system (Celia Brown and Peter Stastny), and by the people behind the first course in Mad history to make it into a university setting (Danielle Landry and Kathryn Church). This section also features survivor (Alison Faulkner, Cath Roper) and allies' (Reima Maglajlic) perspectives on the meaning, hardships and potentials of collaborations.

All of the contributions to this collection raise important questions for the future development of research, theory and social responses to madness and distress. Therefore, instead of enforcing any conclusions, we invited authors to reflect on what they consider to be the most important issues to take forward in the future. The contributions we received form the closing chapter of this collection. They focus on how we can overcome biomedical psychiatry and connect with one another in new and meaningful ways.

Editing this book has an immense personal meaning for us. Unlike many of our involvement experiences, working on this collection gave us the freedom to think and create together, to our own agenda. Although we worked without financial resources and for hours that threatened to become endless, this work was also a luxury and a privilege. We are happy that we were able to include both published authors and those who are publishing for the first time, or for the first time in English. An important learning point for future editors of such international collections is the need for resources for translation. We regret that we could not invite many more contributions and hope this book will inspire future collections of this kind. We warmly thank all the contributors for the time and the work they invested in this collection. We are also grateful to Heather Allan from PCCS Books for believing in this project and supporting it from the beginning and to Catherine Jackson for her tender, patient and professional copy editing.

Before we invite you on a reading journey, let us briefly come back to the very beginning: the welcome note to the conference that is the foundation of this book. Written by Debra Shulkes on behalf of the European Network of (ex)Users and Survivors of Psychiatry, the welcome note reminded us of the metaphor used in the conference and book title:

We do not accept the answer delivered famously by the psychiatrist character in Joanne Greenberg's semi-autobiographical novel that we were not 'promised a rose garden'. The determination of the global user/survivor movement to grow and safeguard this garden ourselves is evident in its extraordinary negotiation efforts leading to the adoption of the United Nations Convention on the Rights of People with Disabilities in 2006.

Our search for a rose garden that was never promised to us is neither complete nor finished, and it might not even be a destination we wish to reach. The main value of the rose garden might be our right to search for it ourselves, collectively and regardless of anyone's promises. That right cannot be denied to people labelled mad anymore.

References

LeFrançois B, Menzies R, Reaume G (eds) (2013). *Mad Matters: a critical reader in Canadian Mad Studies*. Toronto: Canadian Scholars' Press.

SETTING THE SCENE

1

Responses to a legacy of harm

Mary O'Hagan

When I first encountered psychiatry as a young woman I believed the psychiatrists and nurses could help me. I thought they would understand my monumental struggle and give me wise advice on how to live through it. I thought the pills would help to correct the chemical imbalance they told me about. I didn't trust them easily but I believed they had the tools to help me get better. Since that day, over 30 years ago, my belief in the good of psychiatry has been gradually eroded, first by my personal experience, then by learning about the experiences of many others, then by learning about psychiatry itself.

I'm thankful I wasn't profoundly harmed by psychiatry. I wasn't subjected to forced treatment, locked up or treated cruelly, though I came perilously close. Most of the professionals I came across tried to do their best. It was not so much their harm but their failure to help that started my disillusionment – their inability to understand my experiences, their view of me as a bundle of deficits, their pessimism about my future and their failure to offer much beyond 'meds and beds'. I spent nine impossible years cycling in and out of psychiatrists' offices and hospitals. After a few years I began to ask some very reasonable questions about the efficacy of psychiatry. Why is it called an illness? Why don't the drugs work? How can I learn to live with my mood swings instead of against them? The professionals never answered my questions front on; some did not appear to even understand them.

So I read books by Szasz, Foucault and Laing that questioned the biological underpinning of psychiatry, exposed its terrible legacy as an agent of control and criticised the widespread use of drugs. I found out that the nature of 'mental illness' and our society's responses to it are highly contested. I approached my reading with the same scepticism I applied to psychiatry but it opened up the possibility that the psychiatrists' interpretation of my experiences were deeply flawed. Then I discovered by accident a seminal book by an American called Judi Chamberlin, who was a pioneer in the 'mad movement'. *On Our Own* (Chamberlin, 1978) was not an ivory tower critique but one based on lived experience of receiving services. Chamberlin's treatment was worse than mine but her arguments against the medical model and forced treatment resonated with me, and her assertion that people with lived experience should be self-determining and can run their own services was a revelation that changed my life.

In the meantime, after many years, I was given an antidepressant that appeared to work for me and facilitated my exit from the mental health system. Although I remained critical of psychiatry, I now believed I had something to thank it for.

The next big wave of disillusionment came during my initial years working in the mad movement when I read and listened to hundreds of people's stories of their experiences of receiving mental health services in many parts of the world. These stories came through conversations, my research, published memoirs and 'mad movement' literature. Their experiences of harm were almost ubiquitous: they talked of institutionalisation, forced treatment, pessimistic prognoses, cruelty or social stigma that diminished their personhood. Some of the people who told their stories were activists who had a framework for resistance, but many of them lacked any coherent critique – their stories of harm were implied or framed as something they deserved or accepted as inevitable. Many people had experienced kindness and good treatment as well, but they were occasional bright spots in a bleak landscape.

During those early years I worked as a peer supporter and peer advocate inside a large psychiatric hospital in New Zealand that was preparing for closure. I had always believed that the people who treated me, with all their limitations, were looking out for my interests, and perhaps they were. But I became deeply disillusioned by the rampant professional self-interest that dominated the discourse and decision-making within the hospital. The nurses as a group seemed to be far more interested in preserving their pay and conditions than in the welfare of the patients, whom they often neglected and occasionally abused. Some of the doctors behaved like peeved lords who were losing their manor. The management were preoccupied with health board politics, funding or workforce discontent and hardly ever talked about the patients. The staff who cared about the patients often didn't last very long.

The closure of New Zealand's psychiatric hospitals in the 1990s was a big achievement but it did not end psychiatric harm. The locking of acute wards attached to general hospitals, the introduction of compulsory treatment in the community, a growing preoccupation with risk management and supervised accommodation simply shifted the location of psychiatric coercion. But around this time a counterforce to traditional psychiatry was beginning – it was called the recovery movement. It challenged psychiatry to hold hope, respect lived experience and promote self-determination. It called for a reduced focus on deficits and symptom reduction and a greater focus on strengths and connecting people to valued social roles in their communities. We hoped the recovery movement would change the fundamentals of mental health systems. These systems took a while to adopt recovery but typically its impact was diluted as recovery was fitted around the impermeable edges of coercive, medically dominated services. Some people in the mad movement initially rejected recovery, either for semantic reasons or because it was individualistic, or because it lacked a critique of medical and forced interventions; more recently they have rejected recovery because it has been colonised by mental health systems (Morrow, 2013).

Over the next decade I read many books that critiqued the widespread use of psychiatric drugs, starting with Breggin and moving onto Healy, Moncrieff, Kirsch and Whitaker. They all argued that the drugs do not correct a brain imbalance, that they have serious adverse effects, that they do not improve outcomes and that the drug companies put profit before truth and ethics. I considered the likelihood that much of the benefit I experienced from the antidepressants was the placebo effect. I also speculated that my quick return to a comfortable state of mind after reducing or stopping them in the past had been due to the relief of withdrawal symptoms rather than relief of mood symptoms. These books persuaded me to free myself of antidepressants. The withdrawal effects were so distressing it took me two and a half years to get off them.

Over the years I've seen the harmful impact of the psychiatric drugs on many people – tardive dyskinesia, huge weight gain, diabetes, sexual dysfunction and a psychic deadening. I've known people forced indefinitely to take drugs that have the same effects on life expectancy as smoking a packet of cigarettes a day. Most people can access drugs and hospitals (even when they don't consent to them) but no country reliably offers access to talking therapies, peer support, or support in education, employment, housing and day-to-day living. A majority of people who use services have trauma histories that are routinely ignored in the fruitless search for brain diseases and chemical cures (Mauritz et al, 2013).

In a number of Western jurisdictions rates of compulsory detention and treatment are rising to levels not seen since the post-World War 2 era. Most mental health systems allocate less than 10 per cent of funding to non-clinical support services, yet people say these are often most helpful for their personal recovery. Despite the billions that go into mental health systems, outcomes are persistently poor: people who use mental health services die up to 25 years younger than average (Parks et al, 2006); around 80 per cent are unemployed and rely on welfare for their income; and they are much less likely to have a partner or children than other citizens (Morgan et al, 2011).

Over the years I've realised the evidence for traditional Western mental health systems doesn't stack up. An analysis of long-term studies of people with a diagnosis of schizophrenia showed that recovery rates among people with this diagnosis did not improve over the 20th century, despite the advent of antipsychotic drugs and deinstitutionalisation (Warner, 1994). The author concluded that increases in recovery rates over the century were correlated with improved labour market conditions. Two World Health Organisation studies of outcomes for people diagnosed with schizophrenia showed that people in low-income countries with minimal mental health services and psychiatric drugs tended to experience better outcomes than people who used services in high income countries (Jablensky, 1992). There is also evidence from high income countries that taking fewer antipsychotics leads to better outcomes in people diagnosed with schizophrenia (Wunderink, 2013).

Since my first encounter with psychiatry my knowledge of it has broadened and deepened as I have listened to people's stories, travelled the world, worked at the grass roots and led system change. Despite my best attempts to be fair and measured, I have reached the conclusion that psychiatric harm is routine and widespread. It is not something that just happens as a result of poor performance or ethical lapses committed by a few. It is ingrained in the fabric of psychiatry – against a backdrop of community stigma and discrimination – by mental health legislation, narrow funding allocations, Big Pharma, professional vested interests and harmful practices committed by many. After 30 years I know enough to say with some certainty that psychiatry does much more harm than good.

I believe it is more productive to offer an alternative vision rather than to simply critique the status quo. This book will help to foster an alternative vision based on our lived experience. We need a fundamental shift in the way the mental health system and society respond to people with major mental distress.

We need to imagine and create a world where mental distress is viewed primarily through the eyes of the people who experience it – as a legitimate though challenging experience from which value and meaning can be derived.

We need a world where the purpose of mental health services is to support people to lead their own recovery in a milieu that is underpinned by hope, self-determination, a broad choice of services and social inclusion.

We need a world where the culture of services is egalitarian, peer led and community facing; where services are situated in 'natural' community settings; where those in crisis are supported at home or in community houses; where safety is viewed from a lived experience perspective and is achieved by people rather than locks and keys; where there is no special mental health legislation that takes away a person's right to consent; where there is no insanity defence but a humane criminal justice system that considers the broad range of mitigating factors in any crime committed by any person.

I am confident that this book will fill in some of these spaces as it explores peer-led alternatives to psychiatry. However, I am waiting for the day when the ideas and initiatives reported here no longer need to be called alternatives because they have become an integral part of a radically transformed, humane, peer-led mental health system.

References

Chamberlin J (1978). *On Our Own: patient-controlled alternatives to the mental health system.* New York: Haworth Press.

Jablensky A, Sartorius N, Ernberg G, Anker M, Korten A, Cooper JE et al (1992). Schizophrenia: manifestations, incidence and course in different cultures. A World Health Organization ten-country study. *Psychological Medicine Monograph Supplement 20*: 1–97.

Mauritz M, Goossens P, Draijer N, van Achterberg T (2013). Prevalence of interpersonal trauma exposure and trauma-related disorders in severe mental illness. *European Journal of Psychotraumatology 4*: 19985. http://dx.doi.org/10.3402/ejpt.v4i0.19985.

Morrow M (2013). Recovery: progressive paradigm or neoliberal smokescreen? In: LeFrançois B, Menzies R, Reaume G (eds). *Mad Matters: a critical reader in Canadian mad studies.* Toronto: Canadian Scholars Press (pp323–333).

Morgan V, Waterreus A, Jablensky A, Mackinnon A, McGrath J, Carr V et al (2011). *People Living with Psychotic Illness 2010: report on the second Australian national survey.* Canberra: Commonwealth of Australia.

Parks J, Svendsen D, Singer P, Foti MA (2006). *Morbidity and Mortality in People with Serious Mental Illness.* Alexandria VA: National Association of State Mental Health Program Directors (NASMHPD) Medical Directors Council.

Warner R (1994). *Recovery from Schizophrenia: psychiatry and political economy.* London: Routledge.

Wunderink L, Nieboer RM, Wiersma D, Sytema S, Nienhuis FJ (2013). Recovery in remitted first-episode psychosis at 7 years of follow-up of an early dose reduction/discontinuation or maintenance treatment strategy: long-term follow-up of a 2-year randomized clinical trial. *JAMA Psychiatry 70*(9): 913–920.

2

Alternatives or a way of life?

Bhargavi Davar

At a very young age I used to wander around the stale and stinking mental asylums of the 1960s, both those run by the government as well as those run by private agencies, in the south of India. From all those endless visits, I vividly remember my mother being kept tied to her bed, chained to iron bars, or quite zombie-like and in pain with the shock treatments she had received, delivered without anaesthesia or muscle relaxants. These long-term trauma memories, especially the stale smell of mental hospitals, continued with ferocity into my 30s and early 40s, creating havoc on my own mental wellbeing and resulting in crises. In contrast, I also very vividly remember her way of life: her flowing yellow robes; the songs she made and sang about Lord Krishna (a somewhat wayward Hindu deity favoured in most homes); her shaved head (or, alternatively, dreadlocks!), and the many charms she wore that symbolised and protected her celibacy and monkhood. Those were the very reasons why she was labelled 'mad', deserted by my family and incarcerated repeatedly. In Hindu faith, the eldest daughter-in-law had to follow lots of prescriptive traditional behaviours, every one of which my mother violated, favouring instead a life of complete creativity and devotion to what many traditional Hindu households considered to be a sexually brazen male god.

That was her chosen way of life, and not an 'alternative' to psychiatry. Despite her serious mobility impairment, she would escape from those institutions and from our home whenever she could and take refuge in a variety of healing temples in the south of India. Eventually she chose to live in a temple, without any material desires, singing songs to Lord Krishna. I was around 25 years old when I and my brother paid her a final visit in the temple premises, where the temple authorities had given her a room to stay. The walls were covered, end to end and top to bottom, with rather incoherent writings in Tamil. Was she psychotic, and was her florid devotion an expression of the onset of psychosis? Perhaps so, perhaps not…

This is the primary paradox that I have encountered and struggled to understand throughout my working life and through the Bapu Trust.[1] On the one hand in India today there are over 800 'modern' asylums – an oxymoron considering that these asylums use archaic and colonial seclusion principles and other physically restraining, degrading procedures, including solitary confinement. A recent Human Rights Watch report (2014) documents involuntary admission and arbitrary detention in mental hospitals and residential care institutions across India. The colonial vestiges dotting the Indian urban landscapes continue to be houses of horrors, while having an artificial polish of being 'ultra-modern' and even attracting 'medical tourism' within Asia (for example, the wealthy of Nepal intern their relatives in private mental asylums in India, considering these to be 'modern' facilities).

On the other hand, there are tens of thousands of faith-based healing centres in India (Islamic, Christian, Sufi and Hindu) seeking manifestations of spirit possession, black magic, inhabitation by gods and goddesses, arrival of holy spirits and other extraordinary embodied phenomena (Davar & Lohokare, 2008), which hundreds of people visit to be healed or to heal. Several writers have considered ritual efficacy to be an important culturally accepted way of life that does not belong within the frame of Western theory or practice (Sax, 2009; Sood, 2015). Some writers have also argued that even to designate such spaces as 'alternatives' to modernity is an attempt to tie those phenomena to the Western way of categorising human society and processes that may seem alien to Western eyes.

In our study of over 20 faith-based healing centres in western Maharashtra, we interviewed more than 800 people who used these spaces, and they defied categorisation as 'users', 'survivors', 'mentally ill', 'people with mental health problems', 'person with disability' and so on. Mostly they came as 'devotees' to the faith represented by a particular healing centre, with a prayer to be healed from their afflictions. Their 'afflictions' did carry a huge psychosocial and emotional loading, but that was woven into a larger narrative about life purpose, spiritual

---

1. www.baputrust.com

seeking, economic deprivation and social struggles. They diligently followed the rituals, as a family or as a community, in the belief that they would be healed (not 'cured'). Our in-depth interviews showed they were dealing with existential issues, emotionally quite heavy but no less significantly embodied in their manifestation. Of course, they came with powerful stories of estrangement from social development processes, and of deprivation and societal marginalisation. However, a sizeable number of people came from the more socioeconomically stable strata of Indian society, and they were from both the literate and non-literate classes, and from urban and rural areas.

If there was one profound lesson that we learned in these exchanges between 'modern' mental health researchers (a position that we occupied) and people who used faith healing, it was this: attendance at traditional healing centres was a part of the everyday efforts made by the common masses of people of India living in diverse regions and speaking diverse languages to find and nurture wellbeing. To include gods, spirits, angels and demons, *gurus*, saints and other venerable beings in everyday routines and marked by ritual thresholds helped people to deal with their everyday psychosocial issues. This was not an 'alternative' to anything; rather, it was the way that life unfolded for these people on a daily basis.

I encountered 'alternatives' in different ways through my work in the last two decades – through my travels and exchanges with a wide range of people around the world: users and survivors, alternatives practitioners, mental health professionals who advocated alternatives, families who searched for a broader range of support systems than just medication or institutions; researchers and those who occupy global and regional policy spaces. And then there were the spiritual healers themselves, and those who spoke the language of faith healing through the use of a variety of creative arts. These included drumming, song making, possession, artistic symbolisms and rituals that were not cerebral but infused and lit up all the senses. They opened up the imagination and intuition to more nuanced connections between human beings; they belonged to an approach that did not depend primarily upon language and reason.

At a General Assembly of the World Network of Users and Survivors of Psychiatry (WNUSP) in Vejle in 2004, I exchanged news with a global audience of users and survivors interested in Eastern healing techniques. Another exchange I remember was when I was invited to write an article on 'alternative' healing techniques from India for a book. My initial submission contained a section on possession phenomena as a kind of embodied adaptation and healing technique, which is not a new or even a radical idea. However, the editors pushed me to remove that bit because, I was informed, Western readers would find that abhorrent as they associated such matters with superstition, witchcraft and other mumbo-jumbo. I was instructed to keep to the 'evidence base'. Yet, in the last two decades I have in my travels seen that many spiritual healing spaces in India are fully occupied by troubled Westerners seeking spiritual redemption. Nearly all Hindu saints today have a large Western following and vernacular texts are quite commonly interpreted into Western style philosophical writing. I am curious about this overwhelming interest in 'alternatives' in such East/West transactions: there must have been these *ways of life* in the West as well, but there seems to be no cultural memory of them anymore, so people are now moving towards Eastern knowledge and practice, which are sometimes at risk of being adapted to suit Western ways of life.

Can we predict this erasure of cultural memory in India too, and in other low and middle income traditional societies like India? In 2001 there was a fire in an asylum in the south of India, and it became evident that some families were paying a fee to agents for people to be incarcerated as 'mentally ill' in illegal facilities. This led to a national outrage and a renewed dialogue between 'modernity' and 'tradition', with the highest state authorities becoming more prescriptive about the role of faith in healing. Psychiatrists stepped in in a big way at this time, calling such faith healers extortionists who promoted superstition. They raised a clarion call for 'bringing more awareness to ignorant communities' about mental illness and the need for medical treatment. Some state governments set up pilot psychiatric clinics within the precincts of healing shrines, and all devotees visiting the site were screened for 'mental disorders' (Schoonover et al, 2014). While I don't have specific data on these interventions, I suspect that devotees were not invited to give their consent before they were screened or started on psychiatric medication or institutionalised, because *not* asking for consent is generally routine medical practice in India. India is a very patriarchal society, so doctors are revered like gods and mental health doctors take advantage of this reverence by being mysterious about their treatments. Some state governments, such as Maharashtra in the west of India, are promulgating local legislation to 'eradicate superstition' and to make people seek psychiatric treatments. So, slowly in India too increased 'awareness raising' about mental illness is eroding ways of life and bringing about the closure of community healing spaces or allowing psychiatry to occupy those spaces. Some of us who are critical of this over-medicalisation of existential problems are finding it better to advocate for 'alternatives' to psychiatry, as the frame for dialogue has become more restricted and we run the risk of being seen to advocate 'mumbo jumbo' or, worse, being seen as traditionalists if we expose the value of faith healing to wellbeing.

The south Asian and south-east Asian belt is the land of powerful healers such as the Buddha and his followers. However, travels in these regions show that even here the world is getting divided into 'psychiatry' and 'alternatives', and there has been some erasure of cultural ways of life. In high income Asian countries like South Korea and China, traditional healing methods are not regarded as belonging within the ambit of *healing* anymore, and people do not consider it 'modern' to be accessing them. Further, it is not uncommon to find that a particular traditional healing method, such as trance drumming, mindfulness practice or shamanism, is being pulled out of its local context, mixed with postmodern psychology and re-packaged into an expensive 'alternative' that may appeal to the more affluent classes of Indian and Asian society.

Having worked as an activist within the worldwide movement of users and survivors of psychiatry, and identifying as a 'survivor' myself, I have to mourn the loss of *ways of life* in my own life and in my country. At a meeting of the World Association for Psychosocial Rehabilitation (WAPR) in Athens in 2004, Mary O'Hagan inspired me by inviting me to resonate with her faith: 'I would rather be tied to a tree than be strapped to a bed and given antipsychotics against my will.' My faith at the time was: 'I would rather be possessed than depressed!' In these lines, I believe, is both a mourning and a yearning for a way of life that got lost in urban, middle-class families. Such ways of life are still available to a diverse variety of people in India, including the rural, pastoral, hill, mountain, tribal and urban villagers (those living in slums). For the rest of us, we make do with fusion cultural practices of breath work, psychics and spirit mediums, drum circles, pilates, qigong, tai chi, veganism, massages, kundalini and an intriguing variety of exotic practices that go into the box of 'alternatives' today in any Indian metropolis.

I do not want to glamorise 'tradition' or the serious poverty that may have resulted in people seeking faith healing over, say, modern medicine. In the slums where the Bapu Trust works, the indigenous healing approaches are still alive. Many women are inhabited (*Hazeri*) by goddesses or spirits (*Jinn*), and provide community support to other people in distress. They can foretell the future, answer queries (oracle), speak in tongues, and take soul flights (in their own experiences). While some of these women may be distressed or otherwise disturbed, others are able to use these experiences as a resource for their own resilience and support for others. It is sometimes difficult for us to figure out whether a person or a family supporting them with unusual experiences is 'psychotic', 'having an extreme state', 'hearing voices', 'has obsessive compulsive disorder' or is having a great time feeling devout and sacred in their ecstatic bodies. In our work using arts-based therapies[2] we have tried to assimilate ritual healing and the aspiration to transcend the human condition with extraordinary powers as a part of our own healing methods.

References

Davar VB, Lohokare M (2008). Recovering from psychosocial traumas: the place of Dargahs in Maharashtra. *Economic and Political Weekly 64*(16): 60–68.

Human Rights Watch (2014). *Treated Worse Than Animals: abuses against women and girls with psychosocial or intellectual disabilities in institutions in India.* Human Rights Watch.

https://www.hrw.org/report/2014/12/03/treated-worse-animals/abuses-against-women-and-girls-psychosocial-or-intellectual (accessed 27 December, 2015).

Sax W (2009). *God as Justice: ritual healing and social justice in the Central Himalayas.* New Delhi: Oxford University Press.

Schoonover J, Lipkin S, Javid M, Rosen A, Solanki M, Shah S, Katz CL (2014). Perceptions of traditional healing in rural Gujarat. *Annals of Global Health 80*(2): 96–102. http://www.sciencedirect.com/science/article/pii/S2214999614000514 (accessed 21 December 2015).

Sood A (2015). Women's rights, human rights and the state: reconfiguring gender and mental health concerns in India. In: Davar BV, Ravindran S (eds). *Gendering Mental Health: knowledges, identities, institutions.* New Delhi: Oxford University Press.

---

2. School of Arts Based Therapies, WCCLF, Pune, India. At http://wcclf.org/

3

The haunting can end: trauma-informed approaches in healing from abuse and adversity

Beth Filson

There is a growing body of research demonstrating the relationship between trauma and madness. The Women, Co-Occurring Disorders and Violence Study (Mockus et al, 2005; Noether et al, 2005)[1] and the Adverse Childhood Experiences Study[2] (Felitti & Anda, 2010) have intersected with what survivors have been documenting for decades: trauma matters. It shapes us. It happens all around us. It destroys some of us, and it is overcome by many of us. To ignore it is to ignore who we are in all our complexity.

So it is with conviction that I say that I never had a mental illness, though many different kinds have been entered in various files and charts with my name on them over the years. A doctor once pointed out to me – in the face of what he considered to be my obvious denial – all the behavioural indicators associated with my particular brand of madness. To him, my self-injury was a 'symptom'; my panic was a 'symptom'; my hearing voices and seeing people who were not there were all 'symptoms'. When he proclaimed, not without disgust, 'You have a mental illness,' I'd responded, 'I thought I had stories to tell.'

---

1. The five-year Women, Co-Occurring Disorders and Violence Study was launched in 1998, sponsored by the US federal agency the Substance Abuse and Mental Health Services Administration (SAMHSA) through its three centres: the Center for Substance Abuse Treatment, the Center for Substance Abuse Prevention, and the Center for Mental Health Services. See www.wcdvs.com/pdfs/ProgramSummary.pdf (accessed 6 November, 2015).

2. The Adverse Childhood Experiences Study is available at www.acestudy.org (accessed 6 November, 2015).

The medicalisation of distress

The thorough medicalisation of distress that has taken place since the 60s, along with the emergence of psychopharmaceuticals, has resulted in severing people in extreme distress from the social, political and interpersonal contexts that so profoundly shape who we are – contexts that describe *what happened to us* rather than *what is wrong with us*. What is revealed in the answers we give is that we are profoundly affected by every aspect of the world we live in (Mead, 2001).

My ensuing battle with that doctor – and, quite frankly, many others along the way – had nothing to do with my 'symptom profile' or which 'diagnostic category' I belonged to. It did have to do with the complete abrogation of my right to be a person in the world with a history; a person trying to make sense out of her life. I was essentially disconnected from any context that could have explained the chaos in and around me. This is what happens when the individual is viewed as the problem, rather than the world the individual lives in. When the actions we take to cope, or adapt, or survive are deprived of meaning, we look – well, *crazy*.

When the medication I was taking made it impossible for me to cry, I refused it. 'Why?' demanded that same doctor. 'Because it won't let me cry.' *Surely,* I thought, *it is right and good for me to cry. It is what one does when one is grieving.* But no one asked me what I was grieving for, or why. How did this doctor interpret my refusal to take the prescribed pills? 'I can't help you if you choose to be miserable.' What I learned about madness is this: whoever has the power determines what it means.

I knew that what I was experiencing made sense, given what had taken place in my life. Even then I understood my reactions as sane responses to an insane world. I was told, 'Whatever else might be going on with you is not relevant – it's your mental illness that matters.' This drove me into a frenzy, for now help was just another perpetrator saying, 'You liked it, you know you did; that wasn't so bad; it's for your own good.' I was diagnosed and described as 'lacking insight' – ensuring that I would never be able to legitimately represent my self or my own experiences.

Framing a different story

Trauma-informed approaches adopt a different orientation; they are built on the question, *'What happened to you?'* This philosophy of care got its foothold in the 1980s and 90s, when the field of traumatic stress began to emerge.[3] The study of

---

3. The Sanctuary Model is available at www.sanctuaryweb.com/Home.aspx (accessed 6 November, 2015).

trauma and its impact provided a new way of thinking about the underlying causes of suffering, and likewise began to reveal that many of the things that brought people into psychiatric care, such as self-injury, substance use, overwhelming despair and more, arise out of the individual's attempt to *survive*.[4]

Let me be clear: had someone asked me at that time, 'What happened to you?', I most likely could not have said. Not for want of this knowledge, but for want of a language that could articulate what I needed to say. My experience had been that words are far too needy, too thin and wasted for an actual story. This is important because, until we are able to use our own words to tell our own stories, the context we find ourselves in – in this case, the psychiatric system – says our stories for us, and usually gets it wrong. In the context of the medical model, the story we learn to say is that we are *ill*. We begin to see ourselves as *ill*. We tell stories of illness, and the psychiatric system and, by extension, society accepts illness as the story of our distress. Being able to tell your own story – not the illness story – sets a new social context – one in which mad people are seen in a new light.

The most telling illustration I have of this occurred in 2003 when I found myself in a hospital Emergency Room once again. I had a chronic medical condition that flared up about once every year. While waiting for the on-call physician, I had been asked to slip into a gown. Despite knowing the routine, I was still terrified. I am always terrified of taking off my shirt and revealing my self-inflicted scars. It did not matter that this admission had to do with a physical health emergency. In all my past encounters, as soon as the doctors and nurses saw the scars littering my arms, everything about me suddenly became suspect. In the course of attempting to deal with my medical issue, I had endured the flat-out hatred and disgust of professionals on seeing the evidence of my self-injury. It did not matter how long ago it had occurred.

When the doctor entered my exam room, the smile on his face flickered momentarily. He took in my arms. I cringed in anticipation of the blunt, sharp questions – and the disdain that always followed. Instead, as he unwound his stethoscope from his neck, he engaged me in usual chitchat, then asked curiously, 'What do you do for a living?' I replied in a shaky voice – not trusting that the question was not some trick – that I trained people who had been psychiatrically identified to provide peer support based on their own life experiences. He paused, began listening to my culprit stomach, then said, 'I bet you have a lot to teach.'

This moment was life saving. The dignity and respect for my past with which this physician acknowledged my experience was one more rare stone laid in the foundation of my re-emerging sense of self. What changed? Me? Not really. It

---

4. See the Women, Co-Occurring Disorders and Violence Study, for example.

was the lens through which I was viewed. Teacher, not mental patient. Teacher, not destroyer.

Trauma-informed approaches begin with an assumption that people who come for services and support have gotten pretty banged up along the way. This assumption is paired with knowledge about trauma's impact on mind, body and spirit. Service systems that are trauma informed make a commitment to doing *no more harm* by recognising the potential for causing first-time trauma or retraumatising those who have already endured so much. This commitment propels a thorough examination of the operating procedures, policies and interventions of the organisation or system to ensure that they do not inadvertently hurt people seeking support.

Trauma-informed approaches reconnect people to the contexts that shape their lives. Now we can begin to make sense out of what heretofore has been considered senseless: how we operate in the world, how we interpret all that is taking place, what we believe, and why. This reconnection helped me formulate answers to the *why* of my own distress. I began to understand my own, and others', trauma narratives as a search for meaning, not a visit back in time to a wasteland.

We all have a source, a wellspring out of which self coalesces. Source is comprised of every aspect of our lives: all of our experiences, the events that have taken place, and how we have made meaning as a result. This construction of meaning is a source of resilience and self-healing. The answers we form to the most basic of all questions, 'Why?', is the first step out of senselessness. The answers – no matter what they are – help us make sense out of our suffering. The answers give us reason; the answers organise our experience. We understand ourselves in relation to the universe, god, one another.

In part, healing happens in the re-storying of our lives.

Walking with ghosts

Survivor knowledge has been instrumental in the creation of trauma-informed approaches (Blanch et al, 2012; Mockus et al, 2005; Prescott, 2001). In 2010 I conducted training for a group of survivors developing a crisis respite programme in Vermont in the US. When I asked for a way to define trauma, one participant replied, after careful consideration: 'Trauma is something that happened to you that still haunts you today… and if it doesn't still haunt you, it sure did for a long, long time.'

Inherent in this definition are the key characteristics of both trauma and healing:

- it is an external event. No one 'traumatises' themselves
- it is subjective. Only the person can say what haunts her
- it is pervasive, inhabiting every corner of one's life
- healing happens. The haunting can end.

Those of us who have been haunted know that the ghosts we walk with do not just represent events we may want to forget, but *also* our personal histories. What I know of my own experience is that I cannot separate trauma from the landscape of my youth, from the history of my family, from the recall of love and the source of my resilience. Trauma-informed approaches tap into this, and thus they tap into our strengths. So that the person who appears the most hopeless, the most helpless – the one most caught in the chaos of profound despair – is in fact a person who has not just learned to survive but has decided to.

References

Blanch A, Filson B, Penney D, with contributions from Cave C (2012). *Engaging Women in Trauma-Informed Peer Support: a guidebook*. Alexandria, VA: National Association of State Mental Health Program Directors Publications. Available at www.nasmhpd.org/content/engaging-women-trauma-informed-peer-support-guidebook-0 (accessed 6 November, 2015).

Felitti VJ, Anda RF (2010). The relationship of adverse childhood experiences to adult medical disease, psychiatric disorders, and sexual behavior: implications for healthcare. In: Lanius R, Vermetten E (eds). *The Hidden Epidemic: the impact of early life trauma on health and disease*. Cambridge: Cambridge University Press (pp77–87).

Filson B (2011). Is anyone really listening? *National Council Magazine 2*: 15. Available at www.thenationalcouncil.org/consulting-best-practices/magazine/ (accessed 6 November, 2015).

Mead S (2001). *Peer Support and Socio-Political Response to Trauma and Abuse*. Bristol, VT: Intentional Peer Support. Available at www.intentionalpeersupport.org/wp-content/uploads/2014/04/Peer-Support-as-a-Socio-Political-Response-to-Trauma-and-Abuse.pdf (accessed 6 November, 2015).

Mockus S, Mars LC, Ovard DG, Mazelis R, Bjelajac P, Grady J, LaClair C, Livingston C, Slavin S, Williams S, McKinney J (2005). Developing consumer/survivor/recovering voice and its impact on services and research: our experience with the SAMHSA Women, Co-Occurring Disorders and Violence Study. *Journal of Community Psychology 33*(4): 513–525.

Noether CD, Finkelstein N, VanDeMark NR, Savage A, Reed BG, Moses DJ (2005). Design strengths and issues of SAMHSA's Women, Co-Occurring Disorders and Violence Study. *Psychiatric Services 56*(10):1233–1236.

Prescott L (2001). *Consumer/Survivor/Recovering Women: a guide for partnership in collaboration*. Prepared for the Women, Co-Occurring Disorders and Violence Study Coordinating Center. New York: Policy Research Associates.

4

The role of survivor knowledge in creating alternatives to psychiatry

Peter Beresford

A conventional distinction drawn in philosophy is between the positivism of the 18th century enlightenment, which assumes the world exists and is scientifically knowable as such, and postmodernism, which challenges such ideas of objective 'reality'. Some philosophers have called this distinction into question and suggested that both views are the result of the same mistaken understanding (Bhaskar, 1989). This chapter, however, is concerned with a related distinction, explored by some of the most oppressed and disempowered people in society. This is the distinction between so-called 'expert' and 'experiential' knowledge. While of course there can be overlaps between the two, here the point to be made is that the longstanding marginalisation of experiential knowledge is now being challenged by mental health service users/survivors and other marginalised groups, and that this may offer some of the greatest hopes for both social and self understanding and policy responses to the difficulties we face as human beings.

A revolutionary social model

I want to start with a true story that had a big impact on me. Some years ago I was at meeting of a UK disabled people's organisation (so in this sense this is not a story about mental health service users/survivors – although in another it is). I was in a small discussion group of disabled people with physical and sensory impairments. Among us was a wheelchair user, a middle-aged woman who spoke in ordinary language and was not an academic. She said:

> *When I first heard about the social model of disability, it was like a light bulb being switched on in my head. I knew things differently after that. I no longer thought it was all my fault.*

Since then I have heard other people talk about the way the social model of disability changed them, their self-understanding and their lives. The social model of disability is both a simple and a complex idea: complex because people have been arguing about it and trying to develop it ever since disabled people first originated it, 40 or so years ago (Thomas, 2007). Crucially, it was created by disabled people and their emerging movement. It grew from these disabled people – predominantly people with physical and sensory impairments: from their experience, their *experiential* knowledge, their *first-hand* understandings, *their* discussions and thinking. Thus it came from them as intellectuals – not a separate elite group of academic intellectuals, but from the collective intellectual contribution of many disabled people as a movement, in their own organisations.

So why has this model been so important to disabled people? I think it is simply because it has fitted with their experience; it has grown from it and helps them to see themselves in relation to themselves and the world in a different way to the way many were originally taught. Disability in the West has long been understood in medicalised individual terms. People are born or become disabled and that is a personal tragedy – it means that because of 'what is wrong' with them, they are not like non-disabled people and cannot live like them, or even sometimes with them, on equal terms. The social model developed by disabled people says something very different. It draws a distinction between impairment and disability. It talks about the impairment or perceived impairment that means the disabled person lacks a limb, for example, or it does not work in the usual way, or they have a sensory or intellectual impairment. But it draws a clear distinction between this and what it calls disability, while also increasingly recognising their complex interactions. It says that disability is the negative, discriminatory, prejudiced social response faced by people with impairments in some societies that means they face barriers and exclusions and hostility and prejudice – not being able to have equal access to education, employment, the environment, to relationships and so on. They argue that this is just as significant as the perceived impairments they have and that, while both are important, there is no reason for the hostility and exclusion they face. These barriers have become central targets for disabled people's campaigning and collective action. Disabled people have also developed a philosophy of independent living that says they should have the personal support they need and equal access in society to live their lives on as equal terms as possible with non-disabled people (Oliver & Barnes, 2012).

Mental health and social approaches

Big questions have been raised about the applicability of the social model of disability to mental health service users/survivors, but that is not the issue under consideration here. I am interested in the social model of disability because it is an idea that:

- comes from the experiential knowledge of disabled people
- has been developed by them in their own emancipatory disability research
- speaks to their lives, aims, rights and hopes
- has been a powerful basis for mobilising them to collective action for political and social change
- has already made a difference in the lives of many disabled people, both in how they see themselves and what they demand for themselves and other disabled people in society
- has major implications for mental health service users/survivors and our activities.

What is interesting is that a comparable alternative model has not been developed by mental health service users/survivors. Yet surely it could be of paramount importance if we are to create alternatives to the psychiatric system?

Some survivors have invested hope in the idea of 'recovery', which has recently come to prominence in policy internationally. Its appeal has lain in its promise that survivors would not be written off as forever useless. However it is essentially based on a medical model and under neoliberal ideology has been used to justify pressuring people off benefits into employment, regardless of its helpfulness.

We know that the psychiatric system, after a century and a half, is still preoccupied with a narrow, medicalised understanding of people, based on an expanding and individualising diagnostic system of explanation. This has resulted in an overly standardised system of over-reliance on drugs and pharmacotherapy administered often crudely and arbitrarily and in institutionalised and institutionalising ways. We also know that many service users/survivors see such a model as unhelpful and damaging (Beresford, Nettle & Perring, 2009). We know from our experience as mental health service users, and from the experiential knowledge that follows from this, that this system is often inadequate, unhelpful and oppressive. We have ideas from our experience and knowledge of how things could and should be different. What is important is harnessing that knowledge and experience, individual and collective, as effectively as possible to move to real alternatives for all of us and those who wish to work to support and help us. The hearing voices movement and the self-harm and eating distress movements have all developed our own ideas, models and approaches, building on such individual and collective experience and knowledge. I should say knowledges, because there are many diverse experiences and they lead us to developing many different knowledges among us as survivors.

Experiential knowledge: a key departure

I believe that we, as survivors, with support from our allies, must advance our knowledges, ideas and theories to bring about a very different future for all. Our experiential knowledge may take many forms, including research. But first I want to highlight some of the longstanding barriers we face, so that we can challenge these more effectively.

Some time ago I began to think about the way in which our experience as psychiatric system survivors, and indeed that of other oppressed groups, and the knowledge arising from it are routinely devalued and discriminated against. I wrote a report to discuss this, which I called *It's Our Lives: a short theory of knowledge, distance and experience* (Beresford, 2003). This was concerned with the development of user knowledge(s) – that is to say, knowledges whose starting point is having direct or lived experience, say as a disabled person, person with learning difficulties, or indeed mental health service user/survivor.

Of course research is not the only way in which we form, develop or accumulate knowledge, both individually and collectively, but it is an important and systematic way of doing this. When we find out things for ourselves, from our own perspectives, on the basis of what concerns us, then we will be advancing *our* understandings, addressing *our* questions and taking forward *our* evidence.

However such experiential knowledge has long been devalued in research, and, indeed, more broadly in policy, practice and learning. As I wrote in the report, the traditional 'positivist' or 'objectivist' approach to research emphasises the need for and possibility of research that is neutral, unbiased and distanced from its subject. The unbiased, value-free position of the researcher is seen as a central tenet of such research. By eliminating the subjectivity of the researcher, the credibility of the research and its findings are maximised, we are told. Research can therefore be replicated by other researchers in similar situations and always offer the same results. Research that does not follow these rules and is not based on this value set tends to be seen as inferior, providing results that are less valid and less reliable.

This of course implicitly devalues experiential knowledge. Yet we know that in ordinary life we actually place a particular value on such firsthand knowledge. Service users' knowledge flies in the face of traditional positivist research values of neutrality, objectivity and distance and is judged inferior to them. Judged by such values, survivors' knowledge has less credibility and legitimacy. This is what has happened historically: less value has been attached to such knowledge; we know that often it has been ignored or marginalised. Meanwhile, the knowledge claims of researchers and others without such direct experience have been seen to be stronger because it is argued that they are not biased in that way.

So if an individual has direct experience of problems like disability, poverty or using the mental health system, if they have experience of oppression and discrimination, what they say is seen as having less value and authority. Because they are seen as 'close to the problem' – it directly affects them – they cannot claim that they are 'neutral', 'objective' and' distant' from it. So, in addition to any discrimination and oppression they may already experience, they are likely to be seen as a less reliable, less valid source of knowledge. They are thus doubly oppressed.

What this effectively means is that, if someone has experience of discrimination and oppression, they can routinely expect to face further discrimination and to be further marginalised by being seen as having less credibility and as a less reliable source of knowledge. This is likely to have the effect of further invalidating people who are already heavily disadvantaged.

For this reason I suggest that it is perhaps time to rethink assumptions about credibility and legitimacy. One assumption that particularly needs to be re-examined is that the *greater* the distance there is between direct experience and its interpretation, the *more* reliable the resulting knowledge is.

It is perhaps time instead to explore the evidence and the theoretical framework for testing out whether, in fact, the *shorter* the distance there is between direct experience and its interpretation (as for example can be offered by user involvement in research and particularly user-controlled research), then the *less* distorted, inaccurate and damaging the resulting knowledge is likely to be.

We should all reflect on this in relation both to our experience, thinking and research and to our day-to-day lives. I have stressed the importance of psychiatric system survivors developing their/our own knowledges. This is because I think this has to be our main concern. We need to find out more about how things are for us, what happens, what is good and bad and what we can and should do about that. I see advancing survivors' knowledge as our primary concern. After all, why should we be particularly concerned to advance the knowledge of other groups, like psychiatrists or managers? They have their agendas and concerns. These are unlikely to be the same as ours. We want to make things different and better for us and people like us and challenge our disempowerment. We want to secure our rights and freedom, extend our opportunities and meet our needs. So the bottom line for us may be – do we simply want to reform psychiatric thinking and are we really confident that we will be able to? Psychiatry has shown itself very capable of resisting such reform over a long time. Or do we want to develop our own thinking, as a basis for change and building alternatives? I am not saying it has to be all one way, but I do think we need to be clear about this and identify our priorities.

User knowledges and research

Mental health service users/survivors in the UK and elsewhere have got involved in research and knowledge production essentially in three ways:

- to try and influence existing conventional research
- to undertake collaborative research with mainstream researchers and their organisations, and
- to develop and take control of their own research as user-controlled/survivor or emancipatory disability research.

If we want to develop our own knowledge, take forward our own ideas and agendas, then I believe we will need to focus particularly on developing the last of these – our own research.

After all, what gains will there necessarily be for us, if, for example, we are merely drawn into traditional research methods, methodologies and processes? Why would it help for mental health service users to be involved in traditionally-focused research funded by pharmaceutical companies and narrowly concerned with the efficacy of different drug therapies when service users highlight many other important and neglected social issues for research?

In the UK some serious concerns have already been expressed that, where user or 'consumer' involvement is required by research funders, it is frequently treated as a 'box ticking' exercise and seen by some researchers more as a nuisance than of any real importance. So there are fundamental ethical and philosophical issues here about how to ensure that the involvement of service users goes beyond tokenism and incorporation and about where we should focus our efforts.

I have long been guided by the wise words of a UK disability activist and singer Ian Stanton, sadly no longer with us. He said to me, always make sure that the things that you do, where you take the initiative as a service user/disabled person, outnumber the things you do in response or reaction to the agenda of services, professionals and policymakers. Wise words, I think.

Making the link with mad studies

This leads me to the newly emerging international domain of 'mad studies'. This is more than a discipline, it is also an area of activism and, in my view, offers the most comprehensive, cogent and promising alternative to psychiatry that has developed in recent times. It does not impose another monolithic theory or ideology on survivors. It is not tied to an unrealistic argument for separatism that leaves us as survivors to battle the enormous political and economic power of psychiatry on our own.

Mad studies has its origins in Canada and, while enthusiasm for the idea has been bubbling for some time, what really brought it to major international attention was the book *Mad Matters,* first published in 2013 (LeFrançois, Menzies & Reaume, 2013). What is particularly important about *Mad Matters* is that it takes us out of the impasse created by the longstanding dominance of medicalised understandings of madness and distress. This book shows that people with direct experience, supportive professionals, academics, educators and researchers can genuinely work together for better mental health support, education, research and understanding, without anyone speaking for anyone else. Thus this book brings together different perspectives and understandings and shows the feasibility of new and equal alliances.

There is now a UK mad studies initiative; its website sets out the goals of this new movement:

Mad Studies is an area of education, scholarship, and analysis about the experiences, history, culture, political organising, narratives, writings and most importantly, the PEOPLE who identify as: Mad; psychiatric survivors; consumers; service users; mentally ill; patients; neuro-diverse; inmates; disabled – to name a few of the 'identity labels' our community may choose to use. Mad Studies has grown out of the long history of consumer/survivor movements organised both locally and internationally. The methods and approaches for research are drawn from other educational fields such as women's studies, queer studies, critical race studies, legal studies, ethnography, auto-ethnography (again, just to name a few). But Mad Studies, right here, right now, is breaking new ground. Together we can cultivate our own theories/ models/concepts/principles/hypotheses and values about how we understand ourselves, or our experiences in relationship to mental health system(s), research and politics.[1]

Already things are happening. In Scotland, Queen Margaret University in Edinburgh has run a Mad People's History course[2] in partnership with the Oor Mad History project,[3] a community initiative run by volunteers that celebrates and records the achievements past and present of the mental health service user movement in the Lothians, which grew out of links with Canadian mad studies. The Social Work Action Network Mental Health Charter[4] is clearly linked with mad studies values and principles and is gaining widespread support. In the midst of policy failure, there is grassroots hope.

Next steps

Mad studies offers a powerful framework and unifying idea for challenging increasing psychiatric dominance. To take forward our struggles as mental health service users/survivors, I think we will be most effective working from within our own organisations, our own places, starting from survivor movements and organisations that we control. This is likely to be much more effective than trying individually to influence the service system and broader politics and entering their spaces on our own. I also want to reiterate the importance of building alliances with others who will work to support us and share our commitment as survivors to advancing our rights and freedoms. We know we have such friends. This of course includes supportive professionals, researchers, managers and

1. http://madstudies2014.wordpress.com/
2. http://www.edinburghcompact.org.uk/mad-peoples-history-identity/
3. http://oormadhistory.blogspot.co.uk/p/what-is-oor-mad-history.html
4. http://www.socialworkfuture.org/attachments/article/370/SWAN%20Mental%20Health%20Charter.pdf

others. But always we must seek to work to challenge the traditional orthodoxies of psychiatry, research and services. We also need to work together in inclusive ways as survivors/service users, to address diversity in all its expressions, in relation to gender, sexuality, ethnicity, belief, culture, age and impairment. We need to ensure that survivors facing particular barriers because, for example, they are held in institutions or within the compulsory provisions of psychiatry, or who have learning difficulties or multiple impairments, are equally included.

These are, however, difficult times. In countries like the UK they seem to be getting worse for groups such as survivors. Two recent developments in the UK really highlight the vital importance of developing and accessing our own inclusive knowledge as a basis for action and change. Mental health service users have come increasingly under attack for claiming welfare benefits; increasing efforts are being made to force them into jobs, any jobs, whatever the potential effect on their mental health. There have been numerous health and social care scandals where groups of service users, including people with learning difficulties, older people and mental health service users, have been subjected to abuse, neglect and ill treatment.

Service users, their organisations, their families and friends and decent practitioners seek to highlight these problems, but in the UK they have incredible difficulty getting heard. The mental health and voluntary organisations that are meant to serve their interests are often at best ambiguous and ambivalent and at worst unhelpful to the service users they are meant to support, because they are concerned about their own interests as service providers and organisations needing state funding and support.

So, in developing alternatives to psychiatry that become the mainstream, our urgent priorities are to:

- prioritise developing our own voices
- develop our own forums and organisations for raising our voices
- develop our own distinct discourses
- develop our own knowledges based on our direct experience, and
- recognise the key role of research and developing our own research, as part of that.

Our search, our mission, is to find that rose garden for us all. And when I say us all, I mean not only survivors, important though that is. Because truly what we are talking about here is the human condition. We will do it through our experience and the knowledge and expertise we have gained from it – and we will do it for *all* human beings. That is the special contribution we can make as survivors – as keepers of our unique lived experience: a basis for shared understanding and change.

References

Beresford P (2003). *It's Our Lives: a short theory of knowledge, distance and experience*. London: Citizen Press in association with Shaping Our Lives.

Beresford P, Nettle M, Perring R (2009). *Towards a Social Model of Madness and Distress? Exploring what service users say*. York: Joseph Rowntree Foundation.

Bhaskar RA (1989). *Reclaiming Reality: a critical introduction to contemporary philosophy*. London: Verso.

LeFrançois BA, Menzies R, Reaume G (eds) (2013). *Mad Matters: a critical reader in Canadian mad studies*. Toronto: Canadian Scholars' Press.

Oliver M, Barnes C (2012). *The New Politics of Disablement*. Basingstoke: Palgrave Macmillan.

Thomas C (2007). *Sociologies of Disability and Illness: contested ideas in disability studies and medical sociology*. Basingstoke: Palgrave Macmillan.

5

The co-optation of survivor knowledge: the danger of substituted values and voice

Darby Penney and Laura Prescott

Movements for social justice by marginalised and oppressed groups often face the challenge of co-optation (more usually called co-option in the UK) by powerful institutions seeking to protect the status quo. Co-optation is a process by which a dominant group attempts to absorb or neutralise a weaker opposition that it believes poses a threat to its continued power. Co-optation can take a variety of forms. Dominant groups may adopt the language of marginalised groups and alter definitions of words over time, until terms like 'empowerment' and 'peer' become empty buzzwords or mean the opposite of what they once meant. The dominant group may selectively embrace parts of the less powerful group's agenda and then water down these ideas so they become non-threatening and ineffective. The dominant group may appropriate the personal narratives of members of the marginalised group and interpret them in ways that diminish their power. The stronger group may imply that they support the rights of the marginalised group while, in fact, working to undermine their goals. In this chapter, we will explore these issues using examples from two projects in which we were personally involved.

Co-optation and the mad movement

Since the 1970s, users and survivors of psychiatry in many countries have organised to protest the inhumane treatment they have experienced from institutionalised psychiatry; to expand and protect their human and civil rights; to end forced treatment and other harmful practices, and to demand the broad availability of freely chosen, compassionate alternatives to mainstream psychiatric treatment for people in extreme mental or emotional states. The efforts of these pioneering groups were based on principles of freedom of choice, voluntariness, equality and the right to self-determination (Chamberlin, 1990).

A particular challenge facing psychiatric survivors is the widespread assumption of incompetence by virtue of their diagnoses. This iatrogenic vulnerability puts them at risk of losing the fundamental right to speak for themselves. Movement leaders insist that anyone who survives psychiatric treatment is uniquely qualified to speak, write and bear witness to those experiences. Increasingly, survivors have demanded a place in policy, practice and research discussions affecting their lives. Adopting a slogan of the South African disability rights movement, survivors continue to call for 'Nothing about us without us!'.

Psychiatric establishments – particularly publicly funded systems in Western nations – have responded in several ways. Some try to defend themselves against the critiques of their practices by claiming that harmful interventions were the work of past generations and that things are 'better' now. Others argue that, while the deprivation of rights and use of forced treatment are perhaps regrettable, these actions are sometimes necessary and effective. During the 1970s–80s, public mental health authorities began to invite representatives of the survivor movement to policy meetings and conferences, although typically not in sufficient numbers to have a real effect on the outcome of discussions. Survivors were usually at a disadvantage in such meetings, being unfamiliar with the policies, practices and unspoken codes of bureaucratic conduct. So, while survivors were invited to the table, their influence was, and frequently still is, minimal.

Naming ourselves/being re-named by others

The way we refer to ourselves and name our experiences reflects our worldview. People who are current or former recipients of mental health services – whether voluntarily or involuntarily – use many different terms to define themselves. These terms have evolved over time, and are different in various parts of the world. In Europe, the term 'users and survivors of psychiatry' is most commonly used. In the US, those involved in early liberation movements referred to themselves as 'ex-inmates', 'psychiatric survivors' or 'ex-patients' (Zinman et al, 1987).

In the 1980s, US public mental health officials began using the word 'consumer' to refer to people who used mental health services. While this shift in terminology was intended to be less 'stigmatising' than words like 'mental patient', it ignored the fact that 'consumer' is a term for someone who chooses to purchase goods and services in a capitalist society. 'Consumer' does not refer to an individual at risk of being taken away in handcuffs by police, injected with powerful drugs against their will and held in a locked ward. By applying this positive-sounding term to people who were generally poor and marginalised, the system whitewashed the reality of their lives and implied that significant progress was being made.

The introduction and subsequent widespread use of the term 'consumer' by the US mental health establishment represented a social and political decontextualisation of survivor lives and identities. Re-naming or misappropriating identities and concepts by dominant groups are key features of co-optation (Coy & Hedden, 2005). The new terms are stripped of their meaning and bear little resemblance to the original descriptors.

More recently, the phrase 'people with lived experience' has become a commonly used euphemism to describe people with psychiatric histories. Its use distances the label from the person: people are described as having an 'experience' of something, rather than 'being' something. This oblique phrase is awkward, heady and unrelated to the historical context of the survivor movement. The phrase also begs the obvious question: 'lived' experience as opposed to what – being deceased? The expression literally makes no sense, as *all* human experience is 'lived'.

As these terms infiltrate the discourse of mental health systems, it becomes harder to identify who people with psychiatric histories are as a group; with this loss of common identity comes the danger of substituted voice. The introduction of the term 'secondary consumer' to refer to family members is a direct challenge to survivor authority, offering a proximal voice in lieu of the voices of psychiatric survivors. It is not a big leap from this to the substitution of our voice altogether.

How 'peer support' morphed into 'peer specialist'

The process through which voluntary, grassroots peer support practices – developed out of necessity by psychiatric survivors – were adapted and adopted to create paid peer staff positions provides an instructive case study of the co-optation of survivor knowledge. Over the past 20 years, jobs with titles like 'peer specialist' have emerged in publicly funded mental health systems in the US and some other Western nations. While there is no single accepted job description, this definition from the Depression and Bipolar Support Alliance (DBSA) is typical in its vagueness: 'A peer specialist is an individual with lived recovery experience who has been trained and certified to help their peers gain hope and move forward in their own recovery' (DBSA, online).

Some see the expansion of paid 'peer' staff positions as a sign of progress: an indication that psychiatry is becoming more open to including the perspectives of service users in the design and delivery of services. Others see this development as a co-optation of survivors' experiential knowledge to benefit public mental health systems, leaving intact the coercive structure of systems that rely on the deprivation of liberty and forced treatment.

In the US, peer support emerged as a grassroots, non-hierarchical approach with origins in the mutual aid and consciousness-raising groups of the 1970s. It arose within an explicitly political context, in reaction to negative experiences of mainstream mental health treatment and dissatisfaction with the limits of the mental patient role. In the medical field, peer support for people with physical conditions like cancer generally focuses on ways to cope with the effects of illness. In contrast, peer support for people with psychiatric histories arose in response to feelings of powerlessness within the mental health system and with activism promoting human and civil rights and alternatives to the medical model. It is an interpersonal process that fosters inner healing and growth within a community of equals. Grassroots peer support is characterised by equitable relationships among people with shared experience, voluntariness; choice, the belief that giving help is also self-healing, empowerment, positive risk-taking, self-awareness and building a sense of community (Chamberlin, 1978).

In the early days, peer support was informal and relatively unstructured. People met in each other's apartments, in church basements, in libraries, but rarely in spaces affiliated with mainstream mental health systems. But during the 1980s and 1990s independent, peer-run, non-profit organisations emerged. Many of these groups were supported by government funding and began to offer more structured peer support. With funding came oversight, and soon state mental health authorities were in a position to define what was meant by 'peer support' in their funding contracts.

This resulted in the need for peer-run organisations to more clearly define the vision, principles and practices of peer support, or risk having it done for them by non-survivor bureaucrats. Shery Mead has pioneered this work, developing an approach called Intentional Peer Support (see Chapter 12). While Intentional Peer Support grew from the informal practices of grassroots peer support, it is a theoretically based, manualised approach with clear goals and a fidelity tool for practitioners. This approach defines peer support as 'a system of giving and receiving help founded on key principles of respect, shared responsibility, and mutual agreement of what is helpful' (Mead, 2003). Intentional Peer Support understands that trauma is central to the experience of emotional distress that often results in psychiatric labelling. It is an explicitly survivor-controlled, non-clinical intervention with primarily intrapersonal and social benefits.

On a parallel path during the 1990s, state mental health authorities began creating jobs in traditional programmes with titles like 'peer specialist', in what could be called the 'peer staff model'. While these jobs are limited to people with psychiatric histories, they are not necessarily conceptualised as providing peer support as defined in the discussion above. These positions also differ from peer support services offered through explicitly peer-run organisations because assignments are made and staff are supervised by non-peers – that is, people who are not survivors – working within traditional medical model service agencies.

One impetus for the development of the peer staff model was a study in Bronx, New York, funded by the National Institute for Mental Health (NIMH) in 1990. The study found that several components of wellbeing were positively affected by the inclusion of peer specialists on intensive case management teams (Felton et al, 1995). Based on the initial findings of this study, the New York State Office of Mental Health established a 'Peer Specialist' civil service title in 1993, the first US state to do so (see more in Chapter 20). Darby Penney (a co-author of this chapter) played a part in this initiative – a role that she now regrets. The civil service title was intended to bring the values and principles of grassroots peer support into paid peer staff roles. However, this focus was not maintained in practice. The peer specialists' ability to keep the focus on these survivor-derived values was often compromised by clinicians and administrators who did not understand or support the principles (Stastny & Brown, 2013).

The peer staff model has spread rapidly in the US since the 1990s. These jobs are generally held by employees with psychiatric histories working in paraprofessional roles in traditional mental health programmes, often performing the same tasks as non-peer staff (Davidson et al, 2012). These peer staff rarely receive training about the principles and practices of grassroots peer support. Peer employees are usually expected to disclose their psychiatric histories and serve as role models for their clients. Job descriptions vary widely: peer staff may provide clinical and para-professional services that are indistinguishable from those provided by non-peer staff, they may serve as clerical staff or van drivers, or they may have relatively undefined roles. Relationships between peer staff and service users are usually hierarchical, in contrast to the horizontal relationships that characterise grassroots peer support.

This development has given rise to peer specialist certification programmes in 38 US states (as of 2014) requiring completion of a state-approved training course, using a state-designed curriculum or one of a number of proprietary training programmes. There are no national standards for peer specialist training, and the length, intensity and content of the courses vary widely. They do not generally include training on the values and principles of grassroots peer support (Kaufman et al, 2014).

The expansion of the peer staff model was accelerated when the US Centers for Medicare and Medicaid Services (CMS) issued a directive in 2007 clarifying conditions under which peer support services could be reimbursed by Medicaid, the US government health insurance for those in poverty. The directive defined 'peer support services' as 'an evidence-based mental health model of care which consists of a qualified peer support provider who assists individuals with their recovery from mental illness and substance use disorders' (Centers for Medicare and Medicaid Services, 2007). This policy clarification spurred an increase in peer specialist services paid for with federal Medicaid funding. At the same time, the directive essentially conflated 'peer support' with the peer staff model, implying that any service provided by a 'qualified peer support provider' was, by definition, 'peer support'. Stastny and Brown (2013: 459) observed: 'It appears that clinical services have come full circle to incorporate peers as providers in interventions that have moved far away from the original transformative role that was envisioned by the empowerment movement.'

It should be noted that the peer staff model has been supported and promoted by many former psychiatric patients, primarily by individuals who identify as 'consumers' and accept the biomedical model of 'mental illness'. These supporters take issue – often heatedly – with survivors who believe that peer specialists illustrate a clear example of the co-optation of survivor knowledge and experience. The reasons why people support the peer staff model may include self-interest (these positions offer paid employment to thousands of ex-patients); a lack of familiarity with the history of the survivor movement and the development of grassroots peer support in a political context; or a sincere belief in the correctness and value of the medical model. However, the preponderance of research finds that peer staff feel ostracised and poorly treated by non-peer staff (Walker & Bryant, 2013). One recent study explicitly found that peer staff working in traditional treatment agencies are 'co-opted', reporting that the employment and supervisory circumstances of peer staff 'can reasonably be construed as a powerful force encouraging acculturation into the cultures of the treatment organizations in which they work' (Alberta & Ploski, 2014: 28).

Who has the authority to speak about survivor experiences?

Is it possible to work in established systems and not be co-opted? This issue was addressed by Laura Prescott (co-author of this chapter) during her involvement in the US federally funded Women, Co-Occurring Disorders and Violence Study (WCDVS), beginning in 1998. The study was primarily an outgrowth of a 1994 national conference entitled 'Dare to Vision', which focused on the high rates of physical and sexual abuse among women in public mental health systems. Throughout the conference and in the related publications that followed, psychiatric survivors testified to the pervasive and frequently unacknowledged violence in their lives. They pointed out how this violence was chronically repeated within psychiatric facilities through the use of restraint, seclusion and other forms of force and coercion. Survivors described how the adaptations they developed to cope with the aftermath of trauma were re-codified as 'symptoms', 'disorders' and 'diseases'. They stated that the long-term, damaging effects of psychiatric interventions required a complete revision of mental health policy and service delivery; policy and practice should be gender specific, trauma informed and survivor centred. To ensure the success of and accountability for these changes, ex-patients insisted on being critical partners and central architects of policy, practice, design, implementation and evaluation (Center for Mental Health Services, 1995).

In response, federal policymakers worked with clinicians, advocates and survivors to create a national research study focusing on women and trauma. A key component was the stated emphasis on strengthening the involvement of consumer/survivor/recovering (CSR) women in order to enhance the quality of the study design and efficacy of implementation (Substance Abuse and Mental Health Services Administration, 1998: 7–8). The 14 study sites and the coordinating centre were expected to demonstrate meaningful CSR involvement and partnerships through all phases of programme design, delivery and evaluation over the five-year study period. Although there was a powerfully articulated commitment to CSR integration, policymakers, clinicians, researchers and other stakeholders struggled to define what that meant and how to proceed.

In the project's first phase, technical assistance teams from the co-ordinating centre met with sites to support them in clarifying their research goals, articulating service intervention models and developing multi-stakeholder teams. This included an ongoing attempt to define who qualified as 'CSR' women, and what was meant by 'involvement' that was measurably 'meaningful'. Quantitative measures seemed insufficient. It also seemed important to determine how the environment was qualitatively changed as a result of survivor involvement.

Sometimes CSRs were not comfortable actively participating in meetings, even when there were several of them present. The reasons were similar to those reported by peers working in traditional mental health systems. These included tokenism, inadequate support and training, not being familiar with the language (such as bureaucratic shorthand, research terms), not being informed about the purpose of projects and meetings, lack of clarity about role expectations, and being unsure about how to speak with people who do not necessarily share their values or experiences (Prescott, 2001a; Prescott, 2001b; Van Tosh et al, 1993). When these barriers were present, survivors frequently did not stay involved very long or, if they attended meetings, did not actively participate. This absence of survivor participation created opportunities for co-optation, as others (non-survivors) articulated the issues from their own perspectives.

While survivors were key to the grant development process, it was a struggle to integrate them in socially valued roles as team members afterwards, when funds were awarded. Because providers, programme directors and researchers were used to seeing CSRs as recipients of services rather than as capable partners, their roles were often undefined or confined to peripheral activities like participating in focus groups. Within this context, women were asked to share their histories and expertise with non-survivors, frequently in exchange for food, vouchers and other nominal stipends. This type of superficial involvement exploited people who were, typically, poor and co-opted their expertise for programmatic gain.

Disclosure: whose knowledge counts?

A major issue that crystallised as the WCDVS project evolved was the number of women with personal histories of violence, serious emotional distress and substance use who chose to remain hidden. These tended to be women in positions of power who were concerned about the impact of public disclosure. Many had worked hard to hide their histories in order to remain credible. While it is essential to respect individual rights to privacy, their choices had a major impact on the attempt to measure CSR involvement and on interpersonal relationships among study participants.

Women who publicly identified as CSRs often felt betrayed by women with similar experiences who remained safely in the closet. Tensions intensified when hidden survivors counted themselves as CSR women, even though they did not represent those points of view publicly. This substitution of experience highlighted the importance of understanding the subtle ways co-optation operates and the need to define whose knowledge counts (Russo & Beresford, 2015).

The impact of hidden survivors was felt structurally when sites and multi-stakeholder teams were asked to demonstrate how CSR women were involved. When asked how they planned to recruit survivors as partners, some sites responded that they already had a majority of CSR women working with them. This seemed curious, when none publicly identified that way. When pressed, some administrators were reluctant to identify CSR women or describe the tasks associated with their involvement, citing the need for privacy protection. Systems and services that do not involve people who are willing to publicly identify as survivors not only leave a clear absence of CSR voice but do little to challenge the status quo.

The federal funding agency initially articulated the importance of a visible, survivor involvement at every level throughout the study. This commitment acknowledged the historical silencing experienced by many CSR women. But, as tension mounted over the issues of CSR voice and role, there was increasing pressure to articulate a more centrist point of view, to encourage survivors to be patient with an elongated process of change.

Questions for further discussion

The experiences of survivors with the WCDVS and with peer specialist jobs highlight some issues for ongoing discussion of co-optation. In these examples, survivor values were undermined and survivor voice was diminished. If survivors are to continue to try to collaborate as partners with policymakers and clinicians, issues of power and privilege need to be clarified and addressed.

We need to reflect on whether it is even possible to collaborate without undermining the fundamental values underlying our movement. For example, can we create peer support positions within the mental health system that embody the principles of mutuality and do not become hierarchical? Would it be easier to maintain these values if peer support services were provided by free-standing, peer-run programmes rather than through paid positions within traditional mental health agencies?

We also need to reflect on and discuss who has the authority to tell survivor history. Who qualifies as a psychiatric survivor? What about the ex-patient who chooses to remain hidden and non-disclosing in order to maintain a position of power? Do they have the authority to tell survivor stories other than their own? As more valued social roles are occupied by survivors, will it affect people's willingness to publicly disclose their experiences of marginality? How do we define the parameters of the discourse, not just be invited as guests? And how do we stop our narratives being taken from us and re-appropriated? Who are the experts and who says so?

We must continue to ask such difficult and essential questions. The psychiatric survivor movement has yet to engage in a comprehensive discussion of the co-optation of survivor knowledge. We hope this preliminary consideration will lead to further exploration and spark efforts to regain control of our collective histories before they become lost.

References

Alberta AJ, Ploski RR (2014). Co-optation of peer support staff: quantitative evidence. *Rehabilitation Process and Outcome 3*: 25–29.

Center for Mental Health Services (1995). *Dare to Vision: shaping the national agenda for women, abuse and mental health services.* Holyoke, MA: Human Resources Association.

Centers for Medicare and Medicaid Services (CMS) (2007). *State Medicaid Directors' Letter #07-011* [Guidance to states interested in peer support services under the Medicaid program]. Baltimore, MD: CMS, Department of Health and Human Services.

Chamberlin J (1990). The ex-patients' movement: where we've been and where we're going. *Journal of Mind and Behavior 11*(3): 323–336.

Chamberlin J (1978). *On Our Own: patient-controlled alternatives to the mental health system.* New York: McGraw-Hill.

Coy PG, Hedeen T (2005). Stage model of social movement co-optation: community mediation in the United States. *The Sociological Quarterly 46*(3): 405–435.

Davidson L, Bellamy C, Guy K, Miller R (2012). Peer support among persons with severe mental illnesses: a review of evidence and experience. *World Psychiatry 11*(2): 123–128.

Depression and Bipolar Support Alliance. *Learn About Peer Specialists.* [Online.] http://www.dbsalliance.org/site/PageServer?pagename=education_training_learn_about_peer_specialists (accessed 14 March, 2015).

Felton CJ, Stastny P, Shern DL, Blanch A, Donahue SA, Knight E, Brown C (1995). Consumers as peer specialists on intensive case management teams: impact on client outcomes. *Psychiatric Services 46*(10): 1037–1044.

Kaufman L, Brooks W, Bellinger J, Steinley-Bumgarner M, Stevens-Manser S (2014). *Peer Specialist Training and Certification Programs: a national overview – 2014 update.* Austin, Texas: Texas Institute for Excellence in Mental Health, University of Texas at Austin.

Mead S (2003). *Defining Peer Support.* Bristol, VT: Intentional Peer Support. http://www.intentionalpeersupport.org/wp-content/uploads/2014/04/Defining-Peer-Support.pdf (accessed 5 November, 2015).

Prescott L (2001a). *Consumer/Survivor/Recovering Women: a guide for partnerships in collaboration.* Delmar, NY: Policy Research Associates.

Prescott L (2001b). Defining the role of consumer-survivors in trauma-informed systems. *New Directions for Mental Health Services 89*: 83–89.

Russo J, Beresford P (2015). Between exclusion and colonisation: seeking a place for mad people's knowledge in academia. *Disability & Society 30*(1): 153–157.

Stastny P, Brown C (2013). Peer specialist: origins, pitfalls and worldwide dissemination. *Vertex 24*(112): 455–459.

Substance Abuse and Mental Health Services Administration (SAMHSA) (1998). *Cooperative Agreement to Study Women with Alcohol, Drug Abuse, Mental Health (ADM) Disorders who have Histories of Violence: guidance for applicants (GfA)*. No. TI-98-004. Rockville, MD: SAMHSA.

Van Tosh L, Finkle M, Hartman B, Lewis C, Plumlee LA, Susko MA (1993). *Working for a Change: employment of consumers/survivors in the design and provision of services for persons who are homeless and mentally disabled*. Rockville, MD: Center for Mental Health Services.

Walker G, Bryant W (2013). Peer support in adult mental health services: a metasynthesis of qualitative findings. *Psychiatric Rehabilitation Journal 36*(1): 28–34.

Zinman S, Harp H, Budd S (eds) (1987). *Reaching Across: mental health clients helping each other*. Sacramento, CA: California Network of Mental Health Clients.

SURVIVOR-PRODUCED KNOWLEDGE

6

The transformative potential of survivor research

Angela Sweeney

In Chapter 4 Peter Beresford describes three ways in which survivors have become involved in research and knowledge production: by influencing conventional research, by conducting research in collaboration with mainstream researchers, and by developing our own research. This chapter focuses on the third of these: survivor research. The aim is to give a short account of survivor research and discuss what it means to me to be a survivor researcher. This will provide some context for the subsequent chapters in this section, which predominantly describe survivor research's contribution to knowledge. We often claim that, collectively, survivor research challenges biomedical psychiatry and represents an alternative discourse. This chapter will also explore the extent to which this claim holds true.

Situating survivor research

Survivor research can be understood as the systematic exploration of issues that are important to survivors from our perspectives and experiences, leading to new knowledges that are transferable between contexts. Crucially, survivor research is based on experiential knowledge, as described by Peter Beresford earlier in this book. Put simply, this means that survivor research centralises our experiences, priorities, perspectives and beliefs about what heals and harms. Many of the chapters in this section are testament to the power and authenticity of conducting research from this 'first person experience' (Webb, 2008). This is in sharp contrast to clinical and academic knowledge, which typically denigrates the knowledge of survivors as anecdotal, subjective and unscientific. However, survivor research in its current form can be seen as dominated by white protagonists, with research by black survivors often lacking funding and recognition (Beresford & Rose, 2009). Although the first review of survivor research (Turner & Beresford, 2005) concluded that a further review from the perspective of black communities was needed, this has still not occurred ten years on. Alongside dedicated funding for research conducted by and with black and other diverse or marginalised survivor communities, it is critical that the work of black researchers is integral to survivor research, rather than being treated as an add-on to the main activities of white researchers. The racism, sexism and homophobia that can manifest in survivor research is echoed in the survivor movement as a whole, as expressed by Gorman et al (2013) in *Mad People of Colour: a manifesto*:

> *We write this manifesto because we know that racism, sexism and oppression circulating in the system are also circulating in the mad movement. Over the years we, and other mad people of color, have been in mad movement spaces – sometimes as organizers, and sometimes as participants. We have been present, vocal, and visible – bringing forward our concerns about racism, about our precarious legal status, about the experiences of working class immigrants, and about the violent and subtle ways that people of color are psychiatrized. Yet each time we speak or write these truths, our perspectives are dismissed or deflected by people who want the mad movement to be white and middle-class.*

Rather than denying that our experiences of psychiatry are diverse and ignoring the ways they intersect with other systems of oppression, we must all confront and interrogate the ways in which we perpetuate those systems – wittingly and unwittingly – both in the survivor movement and within survivor research.

While survivor research occurs internationally, it is the UK that has seen the greatest activity. Here, survivor research has been flourishing for less than 20 years, although its history is longer than this. It can be said to have emerged from the UK survivors' movement, whereby activists wanted to use their research skills to systematically produce knowledge from survivor perspectives (Rose & Beresford, 2009). The past decade has seen the publication of a number of key texts that signify the continued bourgeoning of survivor research, including *The Ethics of Survivor Research* (Faulkner, 2004), *This is Survivor Research* (Sweeney et al, 2009) and *Mental Health Service Users in Research* (Staddon, 2013); all are UK publications.

However, it is the recent emergence of Canadian Mad Studies that has the potential to give survivor research a new focus and energy. Mad Studies can be loosely understood as a body of knowledge being developed by psychiatric survivors, antipsychiatry academics and others that is critical of biomedical psychiatric orthodoxies and encouraging of radical alternatives, and that places the experiences of psychiatric survivors at its core (see LeFrançois, Menzies & Reaume, 2013: 337). If survivor researchers were to develop a strong relationship with the emerging field of Mad Studies, it could provide our work with 1) a new framework through a theorised radical counter-discourse to dominant biomedical psychiatry, and 2) a new justification beyond consumerist service user involvement arguments (Sweeney, in press). In turn, survivor research can offer Mad Studies early thinking around the ethics and means of knowledge generation. Collectively our work has the potential to create new knowledges based on our own experiences that challenge biomedical psychiatry through solid research, advanced theory and radical praxis. The extent to which this potential can become reality will be considered later in this chapter.[1]

Being a survivor researcher

So what does it mean to me to be a survivor researcher? First, many survivor researchers consider themselves activists and are getting involved in research because they want to contribute to change. Adopting the explicit label of survivor researcher is often a political statement meaning that we want to challenge dominant ideas about mental distress and about us. Instead, many (although not all) survivor researchers believe in exploring trauma and social-based understandings of madness and distress, and aim to conduct research that challenges the powerlessness and marginalisation of survivors (see, for example, Beresford, Nettle & Perring, 2010). Thus, survivor research can be an unashamedly political activity. This is mirrored in the work of many Mad Studies scholars who have strong connections to local and national communities of psychiatric survivors and whose work unites activism with scholarship; for instance, Menzies, LeFrançois and Reaume present Mad Studies as an emerging 'field of study and activism' (2013: 3).

Being a survivor researcher also means facing unspoken hostility and discrimination. Currently there are norms around who gets to study whom,

---

1. For more detailed accounts of survivor research see Turner & Beresford (2005), Sweeney (2009), and Russo (2012). To begin exploring the world of Mad Studies, see LeFrançois, Menzies & Reaume (2013), Costa (2014) and the Mad Studies Network (at https://madstudies2014.wordpress.com/ (accessed 3 January, 2016)).

with clinical researchers, social scientists, students and others studying survivors because they are seen to have – or are in the process of acquiring – the necessary clinical and research skills and knowledge. When survivors engage in research, biases against us can emerge, with survivors seen as inherently unable to be scientific, objective and rational (see Peter Beresford's chapter in this book). Moreover, within the positivistic context of mainstream psychiatric research, our approach can easily be misunderstood as anecdotalism or subjectivism. This can directly affect our access to fair peer review, research funding, research positions, and opportunities to develop survivor leadership and capacity, and therefore our ability to establish a body of knowledge.

In the UK, and increasingly elsewhere (for example, Norway), research funding applications must demonstrate service user involvement or justify its absence. This can mean that consultations and collaborations with survivors are experienced by mainstream researchers as a bureaucratic irritation: something that needs to happen to secure funding, but won't – and indeed shouldn't – substantially influence or change the research. Such hostilities are generally unspoken, typically because mainstream researchers feel unable to express these views in the current funding climate and/or feel unable to speak openly against the increased involvement of a marginalised group for fear of being seen as politically incorrect. Nevertheless, these unspoken hostilities can have major consequences for our meaningful involvement in research. Most obviously, the status quo of tokenistic consultations may prevail, contrasting sharply with claims to funders that survivors will influence the research in meaningful ways. More subtly, survivor researchers' approaches to research may clash with mainstream approaches, particularly regarding the role of research participants, yet mainstream approaches may dominate. For example, although equal opportunities for research participation for people from diverse and marginalised communities is an important principle of survivor research, it may not be considered a valid goal by mainstream collaborators. This is because mainstream health services research often prioritises the recruitment of participants who match the demographic profile of users of a particular service. This can limit the extent to which survivors from diverse communities are able to engage with the research.

Survivor research is often based in universities and, while this can bring distinct advantages such as status, infrastructure and access to resources, it can also bring complications (see Jones et al, 2014). Most significantly, academic cultures are often hierarchical, competitive, and driven by neoliberal goals (Beresford & Menzies, 2014). There is a real danger that, by being based in universities, survivor researchers could come to adopt these cultures, because of the pressures of academic life. To combat this, we must hold on to the ethics and values of our practice and extend the same respect, concern and kindness to one another that we extend towards research participants. If we were to find ourselves becoming corrupted by or mimicking academic cultures – for instance, becoming hierarchical, competitive with one another and disconnected from people's lives – there is, arguably, no point in our continuing.

At the same time we must compete for research funding in an environment where service user involvement in research is regarded with sympathy but mainstream research colleagues may not understand survivor research. Inevitably we find ourselves in the uncomfortable position of having to anticipate and address comments from peer reviewers of funding bids without betraying the values and principles of our approaches. Similarly, our written work may be rejected by peer reviewers because it doesn't reflect mainstream research norms. This can mean that we have to revise our written work, implicitly if not explicitly, in response to discriminatory or bemused comments from peer reviewers who do not comprehend the methods, findings and ethos of our studies. This can make for an uneasy academic life. For instance, the following statement comes from an anonymised blind peer review of a paper about mental health service user and staff definitions of continuity of care that I submitted to a journal for publication:

> *Complaining about 'a conceptualization of COC [Continuity of Care] that excludes service users' just doesn't make sense from a scientific point of view. Surely patients and patient needs are at the heart of the COC-concept? Maybe it is politically correct to include service users' opinions, but theory building is not a democratic process.*

Clearly, to the reviewer, service users and survivors cannot participate in knowledge generation or theory building – that privileged world belongs to experts alone.

Being a survivor researcher can mean experiencing the misrepresentation or deletion of our voice. Although I have also experienced trust and self-expression within academic settings, universities and non-survivor research collaborators can feel a nervousness about survivors' perspectives, which creates a desire to control and censor. This is at times driven by the realities of working within neoliberal university settings and the subsequent pressures this places on all academics to secure funding and publish papers. In this context, relinquishing some control of the research design or the content of papers can be hugely challenging, particularly as university employers view the lead academic as carrying sole responsibility for generating grant income and publishing high-impact outputs. However, these pressures on research leaders can have significant consequences for the ways in which survivors, typically the more junior researchers in the team, are able to present ourselves externally, the activities we can engage in and the extent to which final research reports include our understandings of participants' words. Being misrepresented or deleted from research findings can be a particularly painful experience for survivor researchers who have had our accounts of our own experiences dismissed or rejected by mental health services or others throughout our lives (see Cath Roper's chapter for more on the personal impact of working in partnerships).

Finally, Rose has described a 'double identity' challenge that means survivor researchers may be seen as survivors by other researchers and as researchers by other survivors (2004: 29). Perpetually being seen as 'other' can be an isolating and undermining experience. It is therefore vital that we have strong links with other survivors working in research. Survivor research networks can enable us to develop our thinking, advance our methods and approaches to research and strengthen solidarity. Without this we are divisible and consequently far easier to dominate or ignore.

Given all this, why do we do it? Many survivor researchers are motivated by our contacts with psychiatry, which we have often experienced as unable to support us or actively harmful at a time when we are at our most vulnerable. Conducting research is not something we do dispassionately or remotely, or without a significant personal investment. Instead, many of us want to generate knowledge that represents a humane alternative to biomedical psychiatry. But is this really achievable?

Survivor research and the rose garden

As survivor researchers, we tend to explore research themes that are prioritised by our peers. We often claim that this results in knowledge that challenges biomedical psychiatry and collectively represents an alternative discourse. For instance, our research has generated knowledge on our understandings of crisis, madness and distress, the kinds of support that we feel we need and our views on the mainstream responses of psychiatry (eg. Beresford, Nettle & Perring, 2010; Beckett, 2009; Wallcraft, 2002). Many of the chapters in this section provide further examples of the contribution of survivor research to developing knowledge and practice. This building of alternative knowledges to biomedical psychiatry has been a key feature of survivor research since its inception, as evidenced by the following quote from Peter Beresford and Jan Wallcraft (1997: 80):

> *While the findings of orthodox research generally point to incremental changes within the existing paradigm, user-led research posits more radical shifts of control, rights, knowledge and resources to service users and their organisations. It indicates the need to replace the dominant biochemical and genetic research paradigms with more open, equal and holistic approaches. This has led to an increasing interest in and focus on alternatives, to both existing ideas and services.*

Beresford and Wallcraft go on to describe a number of ways in which survivor research challenges dominant biomedical models of madness and distress, including using concepts of distress and crisis; favouring social and spiritual models; understanding unusual experiences as having a number of possible causes; sometimes describing psychiatric treatments as abuse or torture, and seeing medical concepts, language and labels as damaging and inappropriate. The emergence of Mad Studies could strengthen the position of survivor researchers to challenge dominant biomedical psychiatric models as it offers us a unifying theorised counter-discourse to biomedical psychiatry and a focus on radical alternatives that are rooted in survivors' own experiences.

However, a number of factors continue currently to limit our ability to develop alternative knowledges. At present in the UK applications for large research grants often need to demonstrate 'patient benefit' or the potential for service improvements, significantly limiting the types of studies that are considered acceptable. For quantitative studies, funders often expect – and typically demand – primary outcomes such as reduced hospital bed use, decreased symptoms and economic savings, impeding our ability to explore the essence of our approaches. For qualitative studies, funders often require applied output, such as guidelines or tools to support practice. Again, such outputs assume that the research is being conducted in order to improve the current system, and can fail to adequately reflect the essence of our intentions. For survivor researchers, many of the questions we wish to explore lie outside of the current psychiatric system, and our explorations are often at such an early stage that the initial goals are to explore harm and to change attitudes rather than practice. This means that it is challenging, first to demonstrate convincingly that the proposed research represents a problem needing research attention (because of a lack of grounding evidence), and second, to identify direct service improvements or patient benefit beyond iatrogenic and other harm (which is often considered insufficient).

As an example, I am interested in researching whether the psychiatric system prevents people from seeking support while trying to reach out to them because the language it uses is rooted in an illness model that fails to reflect the contexts and complexities of people's lives and how they understand their experiences and distress. The aim of conducting this research would not be to change the language used by psychiatric services in order to increase uptake but rather to expose the large gaps between psychiatric and lay models of madness and distress, challenge the notion that psychiatric models are expert, and explore the validity and credibility of survivor accounts. There are no obvious applied outputs here that would be considered acceptable by most health services research funders.

There are many other barriers to conducting research that present an alternative to biomedical psychiatry and I will briefly touch on some of these. The vast majority of survivor researchers lack the seniority to lead funding bids, and therefore must work under or in partnership with senior researchers who set the tone for the research aims and processes. This, coupled with the need to respond to funding calls and priorities, can mean that our research addresses mainstream rather than radical questions. Moreover, funding for survivor research is rare, and even rarer when the approach challenges accepted psychiatric orthodoxies. This means that even survivors who achieve the seniority to lead funding bids can continue to lack the freedom to explore alternative agendas. A further barrier is that survivor research has strong links with the survivor movement, which has adopted a 'broad church' approach to dissent and difference. This has meant that survivor researchers can be reluctant to conduct research that excludes people who adopt a biomedical model in understanding their distress (Beresford & Wallcraft, 1997).

In his chapter in this book, Terry Simpson describes the difficulties of securing funding for the Sunrise Center, and poses the question, 'What evidence do we have that this process can work?' Many funders want to see evidence before pumping large sums of money into new services. This can lead to a Catch 22 situation where survivors need established services to research in order to generate evidence but need evidence in order to secure funding to establish services. In attempting to navigate the complexities of this, there is a danger that the principles of the new service will be watered down to fit with funding requirements. Mainstream researchers, of course, are able to tack new therapies or services onto existing services, and can explore the differences between the new therapy/service and 'treatment as usual' – a self-perpetuating system.

In finding our rose garden, we need to create opportunities to conduct the research that matters to us. We need to find approaches to demonstrating 'patient benefit' and 'applied outputs' that are consistent with our values and visions. But, more than this, we need survivor researchers and grassroots organisations to work inclusively and in partnership to generate evidence for new forms of practice and knowing. This means making strong links with community survivor-led organisations, seeking paths out of the ivory tower (see Sweeney, in press) and interrogating the ways in which we act to prevent inclusivity. There is hope that we will find our rose garden, but only if we hold on to our values and goals and keep working together to make change happen.

References

Beckett J (2009). A survivor-led evaluation of a survivor-led crisis service. In: Sweeney A, Beresford P, Faulkner A, Nettle M, Rose D (eds). *This is Survivor Research*. Ross-on-Wye: PCCS Books (pp153–154).

Beresford P, Menzies R (2014). Developing partnerships to resist psychiatry within academia. In: Burstow B, Diamond S, LeFrançois B. *Psychiatry Disrupted: theorising resistance and crafting the (r)evolution*. Montreal: McGill-Queen's University Press.

Beresford P, Nettle M, Perring R (2010). *Towards a Social Model of Madness and Distress: exploring what service users say*. York: Joseph Rowntree Foundation.

Beresford P, Rose D (2009). Background. In: Sweeney A, Beresford P, Faulkner A, Nettle M, Rose D (eds). *This is Survivor Research*. Ross-on-Wye: PCCS Books (pp11–21).

Beresford P, Wallcraft J (1997). Psychiatric system survivors and emancipatory research: issues, overlaps and differences. In: Barnes C, Mercer G (eds). *Doing Disability Research*. Leeds: The Disability Press (pp67–87).

Costa L (2014). *Mad Studies – what is it and why you should care*. Retrieved from https://madstudies2014. wordpress.com/2014/10/15/mad-studies-what-it-is-and-why-you-should-care-2/ (accessed 12 May, 2016).

Faulkner A (2004). *The Ethics of Survivor Research: guidelines for the ethical conduct of research carried out by mental health service users and survivors*. Bristol: Policy Press.

Gorman R, Saini A, Tam L, Udegbe O, Usar O (2013). Mad people of colour: a manifesto. *Asylum 20*(4): 27.

Jones N, Harrison J, Aguiar R, Munro L (2014). Transforming research for transformative change in mental health. In: Nelson G, Kloos B, Ornelas J (eds). *Community Psychology and Community Mental Health: towards transformative change*. New York: Oxford University Press (pp351–372).

LeFrançois B, Menzies R, Reaume G (eds) (2013). *Mad Matters: a critical reader in Canadian Mad Studies*. Toronto: Canadian Scholars Press.

Menzies R, LeFrançois B, Reaume G (2013). Introducing Mad Studies. In: LeFrançois B, Menzies R, Reaume G (eds). *Mad Matters: a critical reader in Canadian Mad Studies*. Toronto: Canadian Scholars Press.

Rose D (2004). Telling different stories: user involvement in research. *Research, Policy and Planning 22*(2): 23–30.

Rose D, Beresford P (2009). Introduction. In: Sweeney A, Beresford P, Faulkner A, Nettle M, Rose D (eds). *This is Survivor Research*. Ross-on-Wye: PCCS Books (pp3–10).

Russo J (2012). Survivor-controlled research: a new foundation for thinking about psychiatry and mental health. *Forum: Qualitative Social Research 13*(1): Art 8.

Staddon P (ed) (2013). *Mental Health Service Users in Research: critical sociological perspectives.* Bristol: Policy Press.

Sweeney A (2009). So what is survivor research? In: Sweeney A, Beresford P, Faulkner A, Nettle M, Rose D (eds). *This is Survivor Research.* Ross-on-Wye: PCCS Books (pp22–37).

Sweeney A (in press). Why mad studies needs survivor research and survivor research needs mad studies. *Intersectionalities* 5(2) – special issue on mad studies: intersections with disability studies, social work and 'mental health'.

Sweeney A, Beresford P, Faulkner A, Nettle M, Rose D (eds) (2009). *This is survivor Research.* Ross-on-Wye: PCCS Books.

Turner M, Beresford P (2005). *User-Controlled Research: its meaning and potential.* Eastleigh, Hampshire: INVOLVE.

Wallcraft J (2002). *Turning Towards Recovery? A study of personal narratives of mental health crisis and breakdown.* Unpublished PhD thesis. London: South Bank University.

Webb D (2008). *User-Led Research.* [Online video.] Retrieved from https://vimeo.com/636062 (accessed 13 November, 2015).

7

Towards our own framework, or reclaiming madness part two

Jasna Russo

Some years ago, I wrote a piece called 'Reclaiming Madness' (Russo, 2002) for an anthology of people's answers to the question, 'How do you manage to stay out of the psychiatric system in which you were once a patient?' This was the last piece I published that was solely about my own experiences. Writing some personal accounts helped me rebuild myself after psychiatry and make sense of an experience that had been frightening and unspeakable for a very long time. And although I no longer write autobiographically, my own life is where all my work on madness comes from. This work was only made possible because I found the reasons, the courage and, ultimately, the words to break a deathly silence – the silence imposed on us by expert psychiatric discourse and chemical treatment. Most importantly, I found other people who wanted to hear these complex and unpleasant stories, who were capable of taking them as they were, and who trusted my version of reality even when I couldn't really express it.

The space opened up by these kinds of interactions has become the main focus of my interest; it is something I believe in and am passionate about. On a direct interpersonal level, it is about the kinds of decisive roles that we can take in each other's lives once we do away with a psychiatric understanding of 'help'. But it also applies at another level that goes beyond the 'ways we carry each other' (see Reima Maglajlic's chapter in this book); it concerns our joint reflections on the world we live in and our joint efforts to understand the multitude of worlds we carry in us. Both these fields of work – developing systems of support and generating knowledge – have historically been denied to people labelled mad, mentally ill or disordered. This prohibition extends to the present day, when we are selectively allowed into these fields, preferably as escorts to clinical allies and variously motivated experts. It is therefore still a revolutionary act when we, 'cases to be managed' and 'problems to be solved', take the lead in defining support and generating knowledge about madness.

The incredibly transformative and far-reaching potential of our collective knowledge is no doubt one of the reasons why we continue to be denied spaces and resources for working and theorising on our own. The distinctiveness of what we have to say continues to be re-framed, neutralised and even erased in ever more sophisticated ways. This might give us even more reasons to connect and advance our thinking so that it is less vulnerable to revisions and co-optation of different kinds. This chapter is about my appreciation of – and learning from – other people's published accounts of madness. It is also about realising that our perspectives connect in ways that may lead to our own model or theory.

I speak here not only of personal accounts but of any work about madness produced by people who have been there (and back) and who absolutely resist medical explanations of their experiences. By its very nature, this learning can never be completed. In the course of my PhD, I am planning to further explore how we can start developing together our own theoretical framework and so work towards a much-needed counter-understanding of madness.

There are many constraints on this undertaking, which is self-funded and therefore fairly small-scale. I will not detail these here but only express the hope that there will one day be an international survivor[1] research institute to provide the capacity and resources that this kind of project deserves. In what follows, I want to unpack just a few of the issues that I consider to be important as we set out on the journey towards developing our own model of madness.

Researching madness and the question of 'how'

Madness can be researched in many different ways and from many different perspectives. It has, however, rarely been studied from the perspectives of those labelled mad, and even less often from the standpoint of their shared knowledge. Survivor researchers David Crepaz-Keay and Jayasree Kalathil (2013) observe

---

1. I use the term 'survivor of psychiatry' as a personal preference throughout this chapter. This is not, however, meant to exclude people who identify as mental health service users/consumers or as psychosocially disabled or people who don't identify in any of these ways but have experienced psychiatric Othering in the context of prisons, refugee centres, gender transition, foster care etc.

that much importance has been attached to the issue of the representativeness of our perspectives, an issue which is often 'used to marginalise voices that do not conform'. Meanwhile, the far more pressing question of balance has been neglected. These authors highlight 'the significant task of balancing the overwhelming majority of material written about those who are labelled mad by those who do the labelling and those who study them so that we can see a more balanced whole'. As we work towards achieving that 'more balanced whole', we face other key questions: is it sufficient that we, people who have experienced madness and its treatment, undertake this work ourselves? Do our experiences on their own guarantee that we will disrupt dominant approaches? And, given the many inequalities and injustices inherent in the societies in which we live, how do we ensure that our efforts to achieve balance do not reproduce traditional imbalances grounded in racism, classism, sexism, ableism and other systems of oppression?

My own intensive involvement in research work on mad people's narratives (Russo, forthcoming) has confirmed that, in my view, yes, it is essential that we, people who have been labelled mad, undertake this work ourselves. It is necessary not only so that we can take part in the production of official knowledge about madness and restore our own epistemic existence (Liegghio, 2013); it's also necessary so that we can direct our analyses beyond madness and distress to all other fields of social science from which we are currently wholly absent. In their respective presentations at the 2015 'Making Sense of Mad Studies' conference in Durham,[2] Brenda LeFrançois and Richard Ingram each underlined the importance of this work, which they named 'mad analysis'.

At the same time, there should be no illusions that our experiences of being overwritten and classified will automatically or naturally prevent us from engaging in similar practices ourselves. However much our diverse experiences of marginalisation and oppression inform our thinking, no such experience can excuse us from the labour of developing values and principles to adopt and realise in our work. And, even more importantly, no researcher's identity itself can spare us the ongoing work of carefully figuring out and advancing research methods that can turn these values and principles into practice.

Without a doubt, there are parallels between the experiences that we often have as individuals receiving psychiatric diagnoses and treatment and those we face when we try to have our say in research and policy relating to our lives. On both levels, powerful mechanisms have been at work for centuries. These

---

2. Durham University, 30 September – 1 October 2015; the programme and abstracts are available at https://madstudies2014.wordpress.com/archive/ (accessed 14 February, 2016).

mechanisms devalue not only our personal stories but also our very ability to understand and make meaning of our experiences on our own. They refute our capacity to develop concepts and theories that can stand up to something as overwhelming and diverse as madness.

If we are ever to achieve what disability theorist Mike Oliver (1992) calls an 'emancipatory research paradigm' and start producing 'collective accounts of collective experience' (2009:110), we need to learn how to share the tasks of interpretation and analysis in our work. Unfortunately, there is little existing scholarship that can equip us with guidelines on how to do this. The task ahead of us might actually be about unlearning what we know and are used to. Such a process is certainly complex and multi-layered. Among its tasks are re-defining the division of authority between the 'researcher' and the 'researched' in knowledge production and creating methods that can achieve this; learning how to stop reproducing and reinforcing a 'white, Western Mad subject' (Gorman 2013: 271); disrupting academic spaces that focus on individual careers and competition, and developing a multitude of new 'thinking environments' in and outside of academia. This work is undoubtedly highly challenging, not least because of the many pressures and constraints imposed on survivor-led projects. But, despite all the risks and hardships, I am convinced that we should continue to improve our methods and overall approaches and not shy away from theory building. And if we are ever to work together on developing our own models, there is no way round confronting precisely these kinds of challenges. One way to confront them is by continuing to place demands on ourselves and ensure that we respond to them as best we can in our practice. Because the point here is not just to author another model or theory but to do so in a way that is fundamentally different from the traditional ways of building models and theories of madness. This is where I think the truly transformative potential of our contribution lies.

Undoing the biomedical model

No matter how many times it is reformed, the institution of psychiatry always remains interlocked with other regimes of governance. Upheld by the corporate pharmaceutical industry, the biomedical model of 'mental illness' is one of the world's ruling ideologies. Because of this model, other responses to madness are being wiped out on an increasingly rapid and global scale. Yet the responses that psychiatry replaces are not necessarily any less oppressive in nature (see, for example, the sections on experiences in traditional healing centres in Mental

Disability Advocacy Centre and Mental Health Uganda, 2014; Mental Disability Advocacy Centre and Mental Health Users Network of Zambia, 2014).

Moreover, people labelled mad in the Western world remain profoundly connected to medical explanations, whether they accept or oppose them. Our thinking about madness does not start with a blank slate: it takes place on territory already occupied by a powerful and well-established psychiatric discourse. The extent of this became clear to me several years ago during one pilot study. My task was to investigate people's experiences of their first breakdown, based on their published accounts. The paper resulting from that work was never published but I would like to refer to one of its findings. For the majority of authors, thinking through their first breakdown meant thinking through the first intervention they received. It seems almost like we have to think through the psychiatric intervention first and position ourselves in relation to it, in order to be able to articulate and claim back what happened and who we were before. It is the massive nature of the intervention and the impact it leaves that interfere with a chronological order of things.

An important part of recollecting, understanding and ultimately reclaiming the experience of madness is finding the right words. In this process, we constantly meet psychiatry as a point of reference. As Mary O'Hagan has noted (2014: 16), 'there isn't even a word for patients that doesn't put us in relationship to the system that dominates us'. And even when we stop being patients and start identifying as users or survivors or people with psychosocial disabilities, it takes some extra effort to undo the diagnosis and start to explore the meaning of our experiences beyond the explanations we have been given:

> [W]e grow up internalising our powerlessness to define our own bodies
> and minds without the concepts of madness and sanity [...] Even if we are
> critical, it is almost impossible to conceive that madness might be largely
> a creation of language and theory, developed to suit particular historical
> needs. It might no longer be a useful concept in its current form, but it
> is almost beyond our power to 'unthink' it, hedged around as it is with
> many writings, and a panoply of institutions (Wallcraft, 2009: 136).

For a multitude of reasons, many people adopt biomedical explanations of their states of mind, to various extents. Their reasons may be of a deeply existential and pressing nature and should be understood and respected in that context. This is, however, a different debate to the one about the validity of the notion of 'mental illness'. Leaving aside our individual experiences of the biomedical model, as well as our respective perspectives, all the efforts to adapt, refurbish and enrich the 'illness' model by remaking it into a 'biopsychosocial' model or extending it with cultural, ethnic, spiritual or religious dimensions cannot compensate for the fact that there is no evidence to support the model to begin with. As the chair of the task force responsible for producing *Diagnostic and Statistical Manual of Mental Disorders* (5th edition) (*DSM-5*) explains: 'We've been telling patients for several decades that we are waiting for biomarkers. We're still waiting' (Kupfer, 2013). So, given that the foundations of the biomedical model remain missing, we have two options: we can use the numerous opportunities to assist in improving and amending this model on the basis that the ultimate proof of 'mental illness' will one day be discovered. Or we can go in a very different direction: we can turn our gaze completely away from individual pathologies and outwards to the world we live in; we can join forces far more firmly and outspokenly in order to forge a whole new paradigm.

The role of identity when researching madness

For me, it is becoming increasingly clear that a new paradigm cannot be identity based.

A number of authors have pointed out that, regardless of how we personally choose to identify (or not), we need to move away from creating (and imposing) new groups and categories:

> [R]ather than trying to agree on terms we can all use, let's celebrate, respect, understand and agree to differ from other people's definitions (Pembroke, 2009:6).

> Language can broaden and describe so much better than it can abbreviate and classify. It seems to me that we need more words rather than less to describe experiences (Faulkner, 2002: 7–8).

Abstaining from the notion of a collective identity is hard, if not impossible, for movements that are organised around a particular aspect of oppression and still struggling to establish their distinctive political agenda. In recent times, the traps of 'single issue struggles' (Lorde, 1984:138) have been analysed scrupulously in the context of Mad Studies. I find these analyses eye-opening and extremely helpful. Shaindl Diamond (2013), for example, points to the failures of feminist thinkers to understand the institution of psychiatry and the oppression of psychiatrised women. Ambrose Kirby (2013) criticises the gay liberation movement's focus on the wrongs of a single diagnosis. In relation to trans people, Kirby warns: 'It's not enough to get our identities out of the *DSM*, because somebody else's identity is in there' (p170).

But there have also been convincing calls for the so-called Mad movement to rethink its own mechanisms of exclusion and domination. Rachel Gorman (2013) criticises what she terms 'Mad nationalism' (p270), reminding us that 'Mad' is 'more expansive than psychiatric consumer/survivor identities' (p269). Applying critical race, post-colonial and transnational theoretical approaches, she argues against claims to Mad identity as an essential ontology and highlights 'Mad' in its social and political contexts. Gorman also stresses the impossibility of people of colour adopting a Mad identity, which would only endanger them further and worsen the structural discrimination and legal repercussions they already face. *Mad People of Colour – a manifesto* (Gorman et al, 2013) declares, 'Stop basing your ideas about a collective mad identity on the dominant culture.' These clear words, I think, challenge not only cultural dominance but any attempt to establish and work with the notion of a collective mad identity. How each of us experiences madness as well as how our immediate and larger environments respond to our madness certainly intersect with all the other determinants of our unequal lives. Furthermore, the experience of madness is always a highly personal matter, as Erick Fabris has expressed (2011: 27):

> *The word madness unlocks my story like a key or locks it up like a safe.*
> *It readies the story for interpretations that would dismiss my pretence,*
> *agency and will.*

It is not only that madness cannot serve as a collective identity; I actually doubt whether it can be a personal identity at all because nobody is at all times only mad. I agree with Louise Tam when she suggests that 'madness is something we can have, without identifying as such' (2013: 287); I appreciate the freedom that this stance opens up. Furthermore, insisting on such collective or personal features and enshrining them in our work would also mean preserving the dichotomy of mad and sane. O'Hagan (2014:16) has powerfully described what is wrong with such a division:

> *[I] cannot see the origins of my madness and my sanity as two parallel*
> *stories; they are one story in two dimensions. Madness and sanity are not*
> *two different garments, they are the warp and the weft of the same fabric.*

So what do we, people who have been labelled mad, share if it is not madness? What can connect us at all? One ground potentially is the experience of being labelled, feared and Othered. However, not everyone who has been in the psychiatric system has had this experience. And those who share it may not have experienced the system in the same way, due to their other affiliations and their broader life context. What many of us do share is the fact that we have been through altered states of mind or extreme distress or whatever term we choose to name these experiences. However, not everybody who ends up being treated has experienced these things and also not everybody who experiences these things ends up being treated. And nor does this mean that there is one experience of madness that we all have in common. So the fundamental question remains: can there ever be a genuine and legitimate 'we' that can enable people who have experienced madness to confront the biomedical misinterpretation and appropriation of that experience? Can the broad spectrum of our experiences – woven as they are into different social, economic and political systems – be the grounds for our connection? And can these experiences underwrite our joint work towards a different understanding of madness and the creation of radically different social responses? I am convinced that they not only can but should.

The fact that so many of us have powerfully articulated our own first-person accounts in opposition to the third-person, 'expert' versions makes me believe that this is both possible and worth attempting in the first-person plural. But it will not be enough just to declare such a 'we' or base it on a fragile notion of collective mad identity. Researching and theorising in the first-person plural is an ongoing project; it is something we need to keep learning and keep working at. If we are to stop silencing people and forever producing more minorities within minorities, we need not only to acknowledge our differences but to learn how to work with them. We need to make mistakes and to correct and praise each other's efforts. We need to learn how to keep the bigger picture in mind at all times so that we do not find ourselves counted among the liberatory projects that have failed to do so. This belief that we may be able to disrupt the common pattern might sound delusional, but for many of us this will not be our first experience of being seen as delusional. However suspect and utopian the project of bringing our knowledges together to work on our own framework may seem, it also has the potential to bring us to a far more truthful and comprehensive understanding of madness than those delivered by any single-authored, third-person model or theory so far.

Coming back to the personal

Having made this attempt to think big – maybe too big – I feel like coming back to my own little life. I emigrated to Berlin 24 years ago. This was not planned; I was rather lost and didn't really mean to settle anywhere, especially not in a place where I didn't even speak the language. Although relatively young, I was very broken. With the great support of friends, I pulled together what felt like what was left of me to make a last-minute escape from what had been going on in my life and what had started to happen in the country I considered mine. Then I took the liberty of staying in Berlin for a while, until eventually I began to feel very differently. I am still taking this liberty and I guess this is where my love for Berlin and my weird bond with the city come from.

During my first years here, I couldn't stop exploring the streets. I still remember the graffiti at the top of one huge squat by the Wall: 'The border runs not between nations but between the top and the bottom.' This spoke so well to my migrant life. Recently, looking out from a bus window, I was struck by the changed wording: 'The border runs not between the top and the bottom but between you and me.' This hit me hard as a clear answer to many of my dilemmas. I had been contemplating all of our diverse experiences and the communities to which we belong either because we choose them or because we are already positioned in them by the economic and political geography of this planet. And from here, the return to thinking in terms of 'you and me' didn't feel any smaller; it didn't seem apolitical. On the contrary, this message evoked in me a feeling of responsibility for the things that do depend on us; it reminded me of the power of the relationships we create in whatever we are doing. It reminded me that, in spite of all the overlapping systems of oppression, the irreparable damage they cause and their toxic effects on our capacity to connect beyond ingrained divisions, the creation of a new paradigm for understanding and approaching madness lies in our own hands.

At the end of the day, we have a choice: we can let our differences forever divide us and inhibit the work we do together or we can find a way to embrace them and let them deepen, broaden and enrich the uniqueness of our contribution.

References

American Psychiatric Association (2014). *Diagnostic and Statistical Manual of Mental Disorders* (5th edition). Arlington, VA: APA.

Crepaz-Keay D, Kalathil J (2013). Introduction. In: Kalathil J (ed). *Personal Narratives of Madness*. [Online.] Companion website to Fulford KWM, Davies M, Gipps R, Sadler J, Stanghellini G, Thornton T (eds). *The Oxford Handbook of Philosophy and Psychiatry*. Oxford: Oxford University Press. http://global.oup.com/booksites/content/9780199579563/narratives/ (accessed 27 January, 2016).

Diamond S (2014). Feminist resistance against medication of humanity: integrating knowledge about psychiatric oppression. In: Burstow B, LeFrançois B, Diamond S (eds). *Psychiatry Disrupted: theorizing resistance and crafting the (r)evolution*. Montreal: McGill-Queen's University Press (pp194– 207).

Fabris E (2011). *Tranquil Prisons: chemical incarceration under community treatment orders*. Toronto: University of Toronto Press.

Faulkner A (2002). Introduction. In: Read J (ed). *Something Inside So Strong: strategies for surviving mental distress*. London: Mental Health Foundation.

Gorman R, saini a, Tam L, Udegbe O, Usar O (2013). Mad people of colour – a manifesto. *Asylum: the magazine for democratic psychiatry 20*(4): 27.

Gorman R (2013). Mad nation? thinking through race, class, and mad identity politics. In: LeFrançois B, Menzies R, Reaume G (eds). *Mad Matters: a critical reader in Canadian Mad Studies*. Toronto: Canadian Scholars' Press (pp269-280).

Kirby A (2014). Trans jeopardy/trans resistance. Shaindl Diamond interviews Ambrose Kirby. In: Burstow B, LeFrançois B, Diamond S (eds). *Psychiatry Disrupted: theorizing resistance and crafting the (r)evolution*. Montreal: McGill-Queen's University Press (pp163–176).

Kupfer D (2013). *Chair of DSM-5 Task Force Discusses Future of Mental Health Research*. American Psychiatric Association news release No. 13-33. Available at https://www.madinamerica.com/wp-content/uploads/2013/05/Statement-from-dsm-chair-david-kupfer-md.pdf (accessed 27 January, 2016).

Liegghio M (2013). A denial of being: psychiatrization as epistemic violence. In: LeFrançois B, Menzies R, Reaume G (eds). *Mad Matters: a critical reader in Canadian Mad Studies*. Toronto: Canadian Scholars' Press (pp122-129).

Lorde A (1984). *Sister Outsider: essays and speeches*. New York: The Crossing Press/Traumansburg.

Mental Disability Advocacy Centre and Mental Health Uganda (2014). *'They Don't Consider Me as a Person:' mental health and human rights in Ugandan communities*. Budapest/London: MDAC/MHU. Available at: http://www.mdac.org/sites/mdac.info/files/mental_health_human_rights_in_ugandan_communities.pdf (accessed 14 February 2016).

Mental Disability Advocacy Centre and Mental Health Users Network of Zambia (2014). *Human Rights and Mental Health in Zambia*. Budapest/London: MDAC/MHU. Available at: http://www.mdac.org/en/zambia (accessed 14 February 2016)

O'Hagan M (2014). *Madness Made Me*. Wellington: Open Box.

Oliver M (1992). Changing the social relations of research production. *Disability, Handicap & Society 7*(2): 101–114.

Oliver M (2009). *Understanding Disability: from theory to practice* (2nd edition). Basingstoke: Palgrave Macmillan.

Pembroke L (2009). Mind your language. *Open Mind 156*: 6–9.

Russo J (forthcoming). In dialogue with conventional narrative research in psychiatry and mental health. *Philosophy, Psychiatry & Psychology*.

Russo J (2001). Reclaiming madness. In: Read J (ed). *Something Inside So Strong: strategies for surviving mental distress*. London: Mental Health Foundation (pp36–39).

Tam L (2013). Whither indigenizing the mad movement: theorizing the social relations of race and madness through conviviality. In: LeFrançois B, Menzies R, Reaume G (eds). *Mad Matters: a critical reader in Canadian Mad Studies*. Toronto: Canadian Scholars' Press (pp281–297).

Wallcraft J (2009). From activist to researcher and part-way back. In: Sweeney A, Beresford P, Faulkner A, Nettle M, Rose D (eds). *This is Survivor Research*. Ross-on-Wye: PCCS Books (pp.132–139).

8

Whiteness in psychiatry: the madness of European misdiagnoses

Colin King

> *If any one or more of them, at any time, are inclined to raise their heads to a level with their master or overseer, humanity and their own good requires that they should be punished until they fall into that submissive state which was intended for them to occupy. They have only to be kept in that state, and treated like children to prevent and cure them from running away. (Cartwright, 1851)*

This chapter examines the quotation from Cartwright (1851), using slavery as an analytical framework to argue that new forms of racism can be detected in the performances[1] of white psychiatry in relation to African men.

In the first section I will explore how post-colonial racism in mental health manifests as a lack of awareness of whiteness, which to me represents a form of psychosis in that psychiatry as a profession is unable to see the reality of its impact on African men like me and the suffering we have endured since the time of slavery. I will go on to argue, with Littlewood and Lipsedge (1981) but more forcefully, that this whiteness represents a form of 'cultural schizophrenia' – a state of being out of touch with the reality of the subject under its examination (King, 2007) – which manifests in the diagnosis of 'mental illness' in African

---

1. I use the term 'performance' in the sense intended by Goffman in his 1959 book *The Presentation of Self in Everyday Life*, in which he uses the metaphor of the theatre to argue that that our identity is not a stable, psychological state of being: that we constantly recreate who we are through our interactions with others, and these interactions are like the performances of actors on a stage.

men by European Western psychiatrists. I will end with an explanation of the cultural 'sixth sense' that describes the ability of African men who have been misdiagnosed with 'schizophrenia' to detect this invisible whiteness. I argue that the (mis)diagnosis of African men as 'schizophrenic' by the Eurocentric psychiatric system is itself based on a form of psychosis – a delusion of reality – and it is only when Western psychiatry acknowledges the existence of whiteness embedded within its DNA that this harmful practice becomes evident and can be challenged.

Please note that I use psychiatric terms such as 'schizophrenia', 'mental disorder' and 'diagnosis' here not because I buy into their validity but for precisely the opposite reason: to throw into greater relief the mismatch between the language of white Western psychiatry and the reality of African men.

When whiteness enters the zones of madness

To analyse the impact of post-colonial forms of racism in mental health work is to assess how cultural values and practices influence the diagnosis of African men like me. If you apply Goffman's concept of life as a stage performance (Goffman, 1959), whiteness is revealed as a new form of drapetomania. Cartwright (1851) developed the diagnosis 'drapetomania' to describe a mental illness that caused slaves to run away from their slave masters. It appears the reality of drapetomania is still apparent in today's mental health services in the diagnosis of African men like me with schizophrenia. It is a diagnosis that I have challenged for 37 years and have tried to run away from.

Part of this challenge for me is a resistance to the idea that white philosophy is the central truth; that white philosophy determines the meaning of all realities, regardless of differing or opposing cultures, race and belief systems. Scientific knowledge has failed to address this tension between different cultural perceptions of truth. Understanding this, and having confidence in the truth of one's own experience, are central to challenging the power given to whiteness to define what reality is in mental health and to declare African men like me to be mad.

African men are not thought capable of having a philosophy of mind; the capacity for thought has not been afforded to us. This lack of appreciation of the African body as a thinking entity reveals how whiteness defines me as less than human. Yet the influence of whiteness is invisible in European psychiatry's construction of mental illness in relation to African men. This invisibility of whiteness, its unconscious performance within psychiatry, means it cannot be held accountable for its impact on black men.

Husserl (Farber, 1943) suggests that the process of describing one's experiences allows an examination of how one's own perception of reality, of truth, influences the diagnosis of mental disorder. This, for me, is important to understanding how whiteness influences mental health diagnoses. The unconscious performance of whiteness in mental health work can be evidenced by looking at how the experiences of African men are described in the language of psychiatry. We need to explore how neo-colonial whiteness emerges unconsciously in the linguistic codes of mental illness and the diagnostic frameworks of the *International Classification of Mental and Behavioural Disorders* (*ICD*) and *Diagnostic and Statistical Manual of Mental Disorders* (*DSM*). More importantly, we need to make transparent how the languages and performances of European psychiatry are reflected in their interactions with African men in the setting of a mental health ward.

In this interaction racism and whiteness as a performance has an important cognitive influence that is often invisible to the white eye. Whiteness just seems to exist as a set of behaviours and actions that are never examined. Whiteness defines the norms and it is its unconscious performance that creates the mental disorders that psychiatry ascribes to African men. It is only by making whiteness visible in mental health that we can describe its impact on African men. Frankenberg (1993) suggests whiteness and white actors do have a consciousness of how they construct their world, which is crucial to analysing how this construction shapes the diagnosis of mental disorder in black men. This is giving recognition to 'whiteness' and how it functions in behaviours in the organisational settings where schizophrenia is diagnosed, and the relevance of slavery to the way African men are denied the right to define their reality in the transition into European whiteness.

Uncovering whiteness as a neo-colonial psychosis

This denial of the validity of African men's perception of reality in relation to the diagnosis of schizophrenia in today's mental health wards reflects how their resistance to slavery was presented by slave masters as a mental disorder, as drapetomania, rather than as a resistance to whiteness.

An appreciation of the experiences of African men inside the psychiatric system enables an analysis of how whiteness shapes the African reality. The African experience needs to be acknowledged to ensure that there is not an imbalance towards the European perception of reality, especially in relation to cultural definitions of mental disorder. I am calling for a 're-balance' that starts with an examination of Europe's entry into Africa from the 15th century and the emergence of a mental imperialism that removed African people's right to define their world. The psychological impact of this control can be seen in the thinking, behaviours and values through which whiteness dominates the institutions of Western psychiatry. Whiteness is locked into the DNA of European psychiatry, with the effect that there has been a failure to restore humanity to Africans as valuable, intelligent and resourceful, with the resilience to survive the negative psychological legacy of slavery.

I personally struggle with the European approach to mental illness that is solely dependent on norms defined by the white European male. I consider the term 'schizophrenia' to belong to the descriptive language of whiteness that is linked to slavery through the evolving definitions of behavioural and cultural norms. This evolving understanding of mental disorder has been claimed to be a scientific process from the 18th and 19th centuries.

I consider the diagnosis of 'schizophrenia' to be a construction that represents the historical processes by which African men like me are positioned within the Euro/American imagination as slaves to a system influenced by an inability to see whiteness as a value. This value emerges in the ongoing challenges faced by African men who become entrapped in a classification system that does not recognise African reality. Ladner's (1973) approach to the study of neo-colonial whiteness reveals its inability to understand its unconscious contribution to the post-trauma of slavery. The diagnostic classifications of *ICD* and *DSM* represent how African men are perceived in the eyes of a psychiatric system that enacts the cultural reality of whiteness. Consequently my own diagnosis as a schizophrenic can be located in the cultural reality of European psychiatry that has no representation of me as normal. Eurocentric theories impose on my life a set of beliefs and diagnostic tools that are intrusive features of a classification system that fails to see these patterns of whiteness. *DSM* and *ICD* must be understood philosophically as modern versions of drapetomania as they are linked to the trauma of slavery and the experiences of African men exposed to values that bear no resemblance to their cultural world.

Neo-colonial constructions of mental illness

I consider schizophrenia to be a cultural symptom that is not based on the self-reported experiences of African men, who have had little opportunity to make relevant their cultural heritage as a challenge to *DSM* and *ICD*. I suggest an African classification system has the potential to challenge racism in diagnosis and thereby 'de-schizophrenia' me so I become perceived as human. The challenge is to see how my life as a schizophrenic is constructed through *DSM* and *ICD* as articulations of whiteness in my transitions from Africa to the Caribbean and to Brixton, South London. The ongoing challenge is to force the World Health Organisation to review the rationale for the classification process with regard to the African men.

The revisions of *ICD* have failed to consider the legacy of post-colonialism that has influenced the patterns of race and misdiagnosis during the 1980s. *ICD* was adopted around the world, with a new set of diagnostic codes in which the African experience remained vulnerable to the legacy of the World Health Organisation's culturally blind approach to mental disorder. The legacy of these post-colonial practices emerged in 1948 with the movement of African and Caribbean communities to the UK to occupy the slave beds in the mental health system; beds that I was to occupy in 1977 and on four further occasions.

Littlewood and Lipsedge (1981) similarly suggest that both *ICD* and *DSM* in their definition of schizophrenia do not acknowledge the different perceptions of reality across different cultures. This issue of cultural 'misdiagnosis' in relation to mental health, race and culture reveals the emergence of a Eurocentric construction of mental illness that is rarely analysed in terms of its impact on black men like me.

Neo-colonial whiteness and racism in mental health

Schizophrenia can be investigated through the narratives and performances of whiteness in terms of how African men experience being classified as 'mentally ill'. The experiences of African men diagnosed with mental illness play an important role in understanding how psychiatry operates without naming the ideological power of whiteness. During my career as a schizophrenic I never had the power to challenge the interpretation of symptoms that represented the delusions of whiteness that diagnosed me. My life has been controlled by ideas constructed by whiteness about how I should think and behave that led to becoming a diagnosis.

The latent impact of whiteness can be detected in the *DSM* and *ICD* classification systems that defined the reality of my existence. White male psychiatrists do not question their own cultural symptoms, which allows them to distance themselves from the phenomenon they construct; they fail to see what Rosaldo (1993) calls the 'culture of their truth'. They fail to analyse their European and American science and their unconscious relationship to the diagnosis of schizophrenia. What concerns me most is the emergence of a classification system whose whiteness turns the behaviour of the African into an expression of mental disorder. I am concerned about the effect on the reality of the African constructed by the models of mental illness in which there is no acknowledgement of the subjectivity of whiteness.

I suggest there is a 'cultural autism' operating inside whiteness in its failed attempts to understand the subjective experiences of African men, and that this prevents an examination of how European psychiatry perceives behaviour as a symptom of mental illness. Consequently what is seen as schizophrenia reflects only what is significant for whiteness in psychiatry. The lack of self-analysis to examine the inability of psychiatry to connect with whiteness as a process may contribute towards schizophrenia in African men. The interpretation of schizophrenia should be analysed through the experiences of the psychiatric profession in terms of how whiteness operates in the diagnosis of the 'cultural other'.

Sixth sense – seeing and diagnosing neo-colonial whiteness

Fanon's (1967) notion of 'negrophobia' suggests that the European world conditions the thoughts and behaviour of African men to self-hatred. This became apparent to me as a 17-year-old diagnosed with both schizophrenia and 'manic depression'. I saw in the setting of the Maudsley Hospital[1] features of whiteness that revealed how it re-presents the African experience as a mental disorder within a zone of whiteness.

These zones are made transparent through a cultural sixth sense that is the skill to see and recognise whiteness as a manifestation of post-colonialist behavioural norms. This sixth sense is acquired through personal history – it emerged from my expulsion from school, after being stabbed in the back with a milk bottle, and my transfer to a remand centre and exposure to the court system. It started with being inside the experimental zone of the asylum (Goffman, 1961). Whiteness emerges as your name is read out in the narratives of the social report – words like 'mad', 'anger', 'educationally subnormal' – words that are symbolic of a language of alienation, alongside 'angry father', 'unsupportive mother', 'difficult family'. It emerges in the cold, dispassionate, dehumanising stare of a white elderly magistrate as he recommends a 'psychiatric report'.

The sixth sense is developed further while I'm seated on a bus, chained and handcuffed with other African boys, taken to a prison setting. It emerges as the legacy of slavery is transferred to the modern day psychiatric setting of a prison ward, shut in a cell for 23 hours a day of cultural deprivation and dehumanising experiences, a number written on your shirt.

---

1. The Maudsley is a psychiatric hospital in south-east London.

The sixth sense of whiteness develops as an emotional and conceptual tool to translate the narratives of the prison psychiatrist, the prison doctor and the prison social worker that reveal a shared consensus through the white computerised cortex.

The sixth sense enables me to translate the experiences of being diagnosed as a schizophrenic African patient as a way in which white psychiatrists make sense of their reality. The experiences of African men have the potential to show up whiteness as a form of 'cultural schizophrenia' and to raise it into consciousness at the moments when it is out of cultural reality to the phenomena it attempts to construct.

Whiteness represents the series of narratives, scripts and performances as a historical reflection of its post-colonial past that can be mapped by the African patient when he enters the Maudsley Hospital. Medication and incarceration represent the visible complexity of the power of whiteness in its response to the African patient. These experiences articulate the psychological journey African men make through the manifestations of whiteness in the psychiatric setting of a ward. The injection of haloperidol is the slave master's whip, wielded by the white male psychiatrist, distant from the emotion of this intrusion, leaving me dazed, mortified and controlled. Sixty minutes after being given my medication, I was due to take my first ever examination in my life, O level English, hearing the ghost of Cartwright: 'You are black and you are not intelligent enough to be educated, this is where black men end up.'

I relapsed, angry and controlled by the ECT, lying still, wires sticking out, before being returned to the ward. This was my experience of the metaphor of whiteness as an intrusion, as it is performed within the psychiatric system. I could not walk, speak, eat or go to the toilet for six weeks; I was pinned to the floor and injected with a cocktail; incapacitated, my body became dysmorphic.

These interactions reveal a modern day version of drapetomania: a regime of day-after-day imprisonment in a padded cell, no clothes, no dignity, socialised into the role the 'schizophrenic'. This is the assimilation into neo-colonial whiteness, as the African self-adjusts to the cultural white zone of the ward. The cultural conditions of the ward for the African patient reveal the psychosocial values of the professionals and the environment they create as part of the process, which all contribute to the perceptions that I am and always will be a schizophrenic. The psychological stress of racism faced by African men is part of these ongoing values of a post-colonial past that influences the construction of race and mental disorder.

These experiences capture the phenomena of whiteness as it is used to categorise African men as mentally ill. The experience of the ward setting for

African young men who fail to respond to the behavioural conditioning of whiteness reflects whiteness as a psychosis. The ward meeting represents evidence of my resistance in the court of whiteness, where whiteness as a psychosis is vocalised through the multi-agency professionals in defence of their models and their diagnostic attachment to *DSM* and *ICD*. As the African patient I sit in the cultural chains of whiteness, next to a white social worker reporting back on my life career as a schizophrenic – a hallucination in the eyes of white professionals. I see and recognise the failure of whiteness to recognise that these are delusions that are historically handed down to white professionals in their contact with me. I see their hallucinations of me failing to meet the job specification of white normalcy. These are moments in which white professional psychosis is located in its inability to see beyond the models that carry the seeds of cultural schizophrenia.

References

American Psychiatric Association (2014). *Diagnostic and Statistical Manual of Mental Disorders* (5th edition). Arlington, VA: APA.

Cartwright S (1851). Report on the diseases and peculiarities of the negro race. *DeBow's Review XI*.

Fanon F (1967). *Black Skin, White Mask*. London: Pluto Press.

Frankenberg R (1993). *White Women, Race Matters: the social construction of whiteness*. New York/London: Routledge.

Goffman E (1959). *The Presentation of Self in Everyday Life*. New York: Anchor Books.

Goffman E (1961). *Asylums: essays on the social situation of mental patients and other inmates*. New York: Anchor Books.

Farber M (1943). *The Foundation of Phenomenology: Edmund Husserl and the quest for a rigorous science of philosophy*. New Brunswick/London: Aldine Transaction.

King C (2007). They diagnosed me a schizophrenic when I was just a Gemini: 'the other side of madness'. In: Chung MC, Fulford KWM, Graham G (eds). *Reconceiving Schizophrenia*. Oxford: Oxford University Press (pp11–28).

Ladner J (ed) (1973). *The Death of White Sociology: essays on race and culture*. New York: Vintage Books.

Littlewood R, Lipsedge M (1982). *Aliens and Alienists: ethnic minorities and psychiatry*. Harmondsworth: Penguin Books.

Rosaldo S (1993). *Culture and Truth: the remaking of social analysis* (2nd edition). Baltimore: Beacon Press.

World Health Organisation (1992) *International Classification of Mental and Behavioural Disorders* (10th edition). Geneva: WHO.

9

Deciding to be alive: self-injury and survival

Clare Shaw

I work as a freelance self-injury trainer, researcher and author. In my work, I draw from an academic, professional and activist background – but my most important qualification is the fact that I've lived through the things I write about.

Several years ago, I was asked to develop a course on suicide. I immersed myself in suicide literature and research for a couple of months – not the cheeriest of tasks. But in diving into the pool of literature that surrounds suicide, I was lucky to start with David Webb's book *Thinking About Suicide* (2010). That book changed the topic for me. It reminded me that those of us who have lived with the intention to end our own lives have often subsequently made a conscious decision to be alive.

A decision to be alive. It's a uniquely powerful decision to take. It was a great reminder that, at the core of one of the most painful topics around, there is immense hope and strength, and that in engaging with death we also engage with life: what it means to be alive; what we want from our lives.

The relationship between suicide and self-injury

Suicide and self-injury have historically been presented as one and the same issue. In literature and research, guidelines and strategies and risk assessment procedures, there is a persistent failure to distinguish between the actions that people take to survive – through self-injury – and the actions they take to end their lives – through suicide. There's a deeply-held belief that self-injury is a destructive act – made explicit in language like *self-mutilation* and *self-abuse* and in the assumption that self-injury is something that must be prevented. Consequently, self-injury is often perceived as significant only in terms of the risk of suicide.

It's true that the rate of suicide among people who self-injure is significantly elevated. Research indicates a suicide rate of 2.5 per cent in a sample of people treated in hospital for self-injury – around 60–100 times higher than in the general population (Hawton, Zahl & Weatherall, 2003). However there's a greater statistical overlap between suicide rates and substance use – and we don't tend to confuse getting stoned or drunk with a suicide attempt.

So let's come back to that point implicit in my title: self-injury is about survival. The majority of people who self-injure do so in order to survive. Not die. And, as I've already begun to touch on, while self-injury is about distress and suffering, it's also about hope, strength, choice and self-determination. I am going to describe how this plays out in practice. And in doing that I'm going to make a further point – that experience can be one of the most helpful forms of knowledge. In making that case, I'll lead us towards a sense of how services – and how all of us – can respond helpfully to people who self-injure.

Understanding self-injury

Imagine this. You've had a really crap day – not enough sleep, running late, stressed out, manager on your case, an argument with your partner, unpaid bills. At the end of that day what are the things you do to make yourself feel better. Wine? Cigarette? Cup of tea in front of the telly? Hot bath? Comfort food?

I've told you that I draw directly from my own personal experiences in making sense of self-injury – but that explicit valorisation of personal (or 'first person') accounts over more theoretical or 'third person' knowledge isn't just about me talking directly about my own experiences when I'm delivering training. Everybody – including staff – can consider self-injury from their own, personal or first-person perspective too.

So, let's return to that crap day, and the wine and comfort food, and let's think about which of these strategies are harmful to the self.

It's safe to second guess that many of our common strategies for coping with a stressful day are either actively or potentially harmful to ourselves. Cigarettes. Mindless telly. Alcohol. We all know what it's like to cause harm to ourselves. Self-injury is not some strange, marginal, pathological behaviour. In many ways it is at the heart of how we live; it's what we expect of each other.

This isn't to ignore the fact that self-injury is highly stigmatised. The distance between the immensely negative judgements we make about someone who cuts themselves in a state of great distress and the respect we accord to the managing director who works himself into an early grave with long hours in a stressful occupation couldn't be more marked. As someone who has been subject to a wide range of insulting labels – both inside and outside health services – I know a lot about stigma and its damaging impact.

There's a vast number of ways of causing harm to ourselves, many of which are socially accepted or even encouraged. The term *self-injury*, however, is more usually used to describe actions that cause direct, immediate and deliberate physical harm to the self – for example, cutting, burning, overdosing or ligaturing. By recognising that this narrower category of actions belongs to a wide spectrum of socially sanctioned behaviours, I am suggesting that it's useful to move away from the notion of an 'us' and 'them', to recognise that we all self-harm, and to use this as the most useful starting place for understanding self-injury and how we might most helpfully respond to it. This is a particularly crucial point to make in an area like mental health where the value of subjective experience – the first person account – has been so effectively written out of what we class as valid, or objective, knowledge.

Why listen to the first person?

We need to listen to the first person because an account that focuses solely on statistics often misses subjective experiences like feeling and personal meaning. In the area of self-injury, that's a pretty major omission. So let's bring in the subjective again and go back to you. Why do you use the coping strategy that you use at the end of your crap day? What function does it serve for you?

Common responses might include:

- it calms me down
- it comforts me
- it distracts me
- it's a way of expressing myself
- it makes me feel better
- it gives me a feeling of control
- it brings relief from difficult feelings.

When we silence that sort of subjective material, not only do we omit areas of profound importance – like how it feels to be suicidal, or why people self-injure, or how people experience being diagnosed and treated; we inevitably make mistakes in terms of how we understand people and how we respond to them. We miss the obvious! We come up with accounts of self-injury that bear no relation to what's going on in people's lives.

For example, in my role as a guest lecturer I was marking an essay from a practitioner working with unaccompanied asylum seekers under the age of 18. The practitioner was explaining the self-injury of a young man who had witnessed the murder of his own family and fled on his own across the world only to experience his closest friend being killed in the UK. His self-injury was, she argued, clearly an act of manipulation, rooted in psychoanalytical conflicts.

After six years of using psychiatric services I found out that, years earlier, I had been diagnosed with borderline personality disorder and deemed untreatable.

Theorists interpret self-injury as the symbolic creation of tiny vaginas (Favazza, 1996), or symbolic masturbation (Emerson, 1913) – a form of perversion or masochism. Researchers look to pathology and speculate that self-injury is the result of endorphin addiction (Sandman et al, 2008), or chemical imbalances in the brain that can be treated with opiate-blockers (Shroder, 1996). Support staff assume that self-injury is attention seeking and that the right response is the withdrawal of support. Accident and Emergency staff assume that self-injury is a masochistic act and that injuries can be stitched without anaesthetic. The media portray self-injury as the copycat behaviour of young people in specific subcultures. Ward staff assume that self-injury is an attempt at suicide and that the right response is the removal of all opportunities to harm or kill the self.

The unhelpful theories that surround self-injury are both a consequence and a cause of the marginalisation of our voices. People who self-injure are mad, in the worst way. They almost always end up with a diagnosis of borderline personality disorder, which is the medical way of stating that, for now and forever, this person is, in Louise Pembroke's words (private correspondence) a 'total cunt'. When people are so mad that they attack their own bodies, we should disregard anything they say or think. Shouldn't we?

We have already recognised that of course there's a link between self-injury and suicide, just as of course there's a link between suicide and any other behaviour born in distress. And, of course, when we respond to self-injury in some of the ways I have just described, we increase the possibility that somebody may begin to see suicide as the only viable option. And vice versa: when we respond helpfully, we reduce the risk of suicide. A helpful response *must* be based in a helpful understanding of why someone self-injures. And the most helpful explanation is the one offered by the person, who can, in their own words, explain the personal meaning of the self-injury: its value and functions, precursors and outcomes.

Making sense of self-injury

Survivor accounts tell us that self-injury is a way of preserving and affirming life, often in the presence of intolerable distress. Survivor voices in research tell us that difficult childhood experiences – abuse, neglect, violence, bullying, conflict, lack of support – are common in the histories of people who self-injure. Similar experiences also feature in adulthood. We also hear about profoundly difficult feelings, including overwhelming emotional pain, self-hatred and shame, anger, powerlessness, anxiety and fear, and, conversely, feelings of unreality, numbness or 'deadness'.

It's in this context that self-injury serves some powerful functions, like:

- *relieving feelings/improving mood* – 'Cutting for me releases all the anger and pain and frustration I feel inside' (Brophy, 2006)
- *giving a sense of control/power* – 'When things were happening to me that I had no control over I started hurting myself. This was something that I could control, I could do as much or as little damage as I wanted, it only involved myself. And I could care for the wound afterwards' (National Self Harm Network, 2008)
- *feeling alive/connected* – 'When I feel numb and like I don't really exist, I cause myself harm and it brings this rush that brings you back down to earth' (Brophy, 2006)
- *resolve feelings of guilt and self-hatred* – 'I felt a warm sense of relief, as though all the bad things were flowing out of me, and it made me feel alive, real' (Richardson, 2006)
- *expressing distress and/or communicating a need for support* – 'It's a way of expressing negative feelings about myself that build up inside me. As someone who finds it difficult to put things into words, it can at times be the only way of expressing how I am feeling' (National Self Harm Network, 2008).

Look again at these functions. When you think back to why you use your own coping strategies, I'm certain you'll find an almost perfect overlap there. We all use coping strategies to help us deal with distressing feelings and experiences. And those coping strategies tend to serve similar functions, regardless of the nature of the harm, the level of physical and intellectual ability, the cultural background, the experiences and the diagnosis of the person who is trying to cope. It appears that we're all human after all. So the managing director who chills out with a cigar and a whisky at the end of a tough day can use his own experiences to empathise with the teenager who cuts herself to deal with the terror of homophobic bullying. Distress makes sense when the individual explains it. Coping strategies make sense in the context of distress. Self-injury makes sense when we listen to those with experience. Human experiences make sense when we're willing to draw on our own humanity – to understand each other. And what's more, we can all use our own experiences as a resource for making sense of self-injury. It's not so weird and scary after all. It's not aimed at the destruction of the self: it's a coping strategy, something that enables survival in the face of intolerable feelings and realities.

Responding to self-injury

So how can this inform our responses? The first point to make is that understanding and accepting somebody is not just the first step in constructing a helpful response; it's the very core of that response.

Back to the crap day. Let's imagine that, at the end of that day, when you're about to turn to that one thing you most want to do to make yourself feel better, someone comes along and says, 'No. You are not permitted. I do not approve!' How do you feel? Frustrated, angry, upset, powerless, disrespected, alone, worse? And how do you react? By getting aggressive, withdrawing, doing it anyway, doing it worse?

Not having our feelings, needs and experiences recognised and accepted is always difficult and is often damaging. Being subjected to room searches, even strip-searches, having our personal possessions removed, being physically restrained by five staff, being locked up for months or even years at a time, being constantly observed, even on the loo or in the bath, being medicated to the point that it's hard to speak or move – these experiences are damaging too. In a service or a relationship that is about supporting someone in distress, such a failure to understand is never helpful, and the outcome for staff and client cannot be positive.

In a context where someone is self-injuring as a way of trying to cope with difficult feelings and possibly to avert suicide, preventing self-injury – removing choice, control, and a powerful coping strategy from that person at their time of greatest need – can be problematic, to say the least. In some cases, it can be lethal.

What does work then?

This is where you get the good news and the bad news. The bad news is – there is no blueprint. The good news is – it isn't rocket science.

After six years in and out of psychiatric hospital, I'm fairly well placed to talk about what was unhelpful about those services. But it's also important to name what was useful. This, in short, came down to individual members of staff and, more specifically, to their attitudes. There were several staff who were helpful in different ways at different times, but two who exemplified everything that was helpful. They were both nursing auxiliaries; so it wasn't about professional qualifications. It was about basic human qualities. It was about the fact that they were warm, caring and friendly. They spent time with me. They took the time to talk to me and listen to me. They helped me to feel liked, cared about, valued; someone worth making an effort to engage with; possible to engage with. At those very dark times in my life, whether in services, among peers or in my own personal support networks, human relationships founded on care, concern, and the desire to understand are what mattered most of all.

It would be foolish to deny that supporting someone who self-injures can be extremely demanding, frightening and frustrating. It can throw up a whole range of dilemmas and challenges and it's worth checking out what resources – practical and theoretical – are available to support you in that. But understanding and working helpfully with self-injury begins with the self. It begins with your own humanity, and the fact that your humanity and the relationships you create are the very best resources you can draw from. It begins with listening, caring and being willing to learn. Every approach and every theory should be measured by this standard – by the simple truth that you make the most difference 'by being accepting and supportive, listening and taking seriously the person's experience and needs' (Arnold, 1995).

Beyond survival

And on that point of hope – your own capacity to make a huge difference – let's return to the point of hope that we started out with. Self-injury is about survival. I self-injured for at least 20 years because it kept me alive and intact; it allowed me to function as myself.

But it came at a cost, not least the physical damage to myself. Probably the highest cost that I paid was the slice of my life that I spent as a psychiatric patient. Six years of spending time in and out of psychiatric hospitals is hard to summarise: fear, [, boredom and powerlessness, alongside the distress and despair that took me into the system in the first place. In that context my self-injury and my eating disorder escalated to life-threatening proportions, both despite and because of the restrictions placed on the coping strategies that had kept me going for years. I felt – and I was told – that there was no hope, and it was hard to maintain any sense of myself as someone defined by anything other than pain.

Yet something unnameable kept me going throughout that time. Even in times of intense distress, I still engaged with life. But in the summer of 1998, at the age of 25, I became determined to end my life. It's possible that the medication I was on played a role in taking me to that place – a week on the antidepressant Seroxat left me elated, uninhibited, cripplingly anxious and determinedly suicidal – a lethal mix.

Certainly the chaotic and dangerous wards on which I was detained played a part. And all this on top of at least 16 years of struggle. Suicidal thoughts and fantasies, alongside severe self-injury, had formed such an important part of my life for so long that it's very hard to state categorically when or how I entered into a suicidal state. What I do remember is that, even at the time, I was aware of a qualitative difference in how I felt. I fully intended to bring about my own death. There was no ambiguity, no lingering sense that I might survive or that a suicide attempt might bring about the change I desired. I wanted out. While still anguished, I felt calm. At times I was elated and euphoric. And, most crucially, I stopped self-injuring.

There was no longer any point. Self-injury to me represented the struggle to be alive.

I made the decision not to die, and not long after that I made the decision to be alive. I stopped struggling to survive and began to struggle for a life worth living – a process that involved change in every area of my life, and which was supported by the love, understanding, care and sheer persistence of people who cared about me. It's an ongoing struggle. But, although I still think about self-injury at times, it's no longer a struggle that's fought at the level of injury.

In the presence of self-injury, you are undeniably in the presence of distress. But you are also in the presence of hope. Someone is fighting to survive. With courage, and meaning, and determination. Someone is in distress, yes, but is fighting to deal with that distress, to make sense of it, to find a way to express their needs. Someone is doing their level best to get through the night; someone is trying to pull themselves out of a nightmare; someone is trying to forget; someone is holding on tight to a sense of themselves; someone is listening to themselves in a language they understand; someone is calling for help; someone is giving in; someone is taking a break; someone is making themselves safe; someone is reconnecting with life; someone is trying to switch off; someone is staying in control; someone is doing the only thing that will make them feel better; someone is telling you who they are; someone is taking good care of themselves; someone is pushing it as far as they can; someone is seeking care; someone is making a statement that can't be ignored; someone is trying their hardest to do what's best for their kids. Someone is telling their story.

Someone is surviving.

Someone is surviving.

References

Arnold L (1995). *Women and Self-Injury: a survey of 76 women. A report on women's experience of self-injury and their views on service provision.* Bristol: Bristol Crisis Service for Women.

Brophy M (2006). *Truth Hurts: report of the National Inquiry into Self-harm among Young People.* London: Camelot Foundation/Mental Health Foundation.

Emerson LE (1913). The case of Miss A: a preliminary report of a psychoanalysis study and treatment of a case of self-mutilation. *Psychoanalytical Review 1*: 41–54.

Favazza A (1996). *Bodies Under Siege: self-mutilation in culture and psychiatry* (2nd edition). Baltimore: John Hopkins University Press.

Hawton K, Zahl D, Weatherall R (2003). Suicide following deliberate self-injury: long-term follow-up of patients who presented to a general hospital. *British Journal of Psychiatry 182*: 537–542.

National Self Harm Network (2008). *What is Self Harm?* [Online.] http://www.nshn.co.uk/downloads/What_is_self_harm.pdf (accessed 26 February, 2013).

Richardson C (2006; updated 2012). *The Truth about Self-Harm for Young People and their Friends and Families.* London: Camelot Foundation/Mental Health Foundation. http://www.mentalhealth.org.uk/content/assets/pdf/publications/truth_about_self-harm_new_brand.pdf (accessed 28 October, 2015).

Sandman CA, Touchette PE, Marion SD, Chicz-DeMet A (2008). The role of proopiomelanocortin (POMC) in sequentially dependent self-injurious behavior. *Developmental Psychobiology 50*: 680–689.

Schroder SR (1996). Dopaminergic mechanisms in self-injury. *Psychology in Mental Retardation and Developmental Disabilities 22*(2): 3–10.

Webb D (2010). *Thinking about Suicide.* Ross-on-Wye: PCCS Books.

10

Thinking (differently) about suicide

David Webb

Stories are important because they are the main way that we share our personal thoughts and feelings with others. But storytelling is more than just giving others a window to the silent, invisible interiors of our subjectively felt experiences. In order to tell our stories we must first *find* our voice, which requires that we reflect on our experiences and, as best we can, make some sense of them. Only then can the words – or the music, the paintings or the dance – be expressed and shared with others.

The story I want to tell is not one about my own personal experience of persistent suicidal feelings, though this will be mentioned occasionally. Rather, the story I want to tell is of my enquiry into suicide after I stopped being actively suicidal in the late 1990s. This story is one of looking back on my unexpected survival in order to try and make sense of what I went through. It is also a story that investigates not only my own personal thinking about suicide but also what the society I live in thinks about suicide. In particular, my story investigates the academic discipline known as 'suicidology' – ie. what the experts in suicide prevention think about suicide.

Suicidology – a survivor perspective

When I first looked at the literature of suicidology I struggled to find my own experience of being suicidal in this vast database of expert knowledge on suicide.

I found myself thinking that, whoever all these experts were talking about, it was certainly not me, and I wondered whether my personal experience of suicidal feelings was somehow uniquely peculiar to me. I didn't think so then and I still don't think so these days – possibly even more so. As I continued to wade through this literature, I realised that the actual suicidal person was remarkably absent from all this expert knowledge. It was as though these experts were looking at people like me through the wrong end of their telescope so that we were little more than almost invisible dots on the distant horizon.

The suicidal urge to die only passed for me when I finally attended to the spiritual crisis that lay at its heart, so I was looking in the literature of suicidology for any discussion of spirituality. I guess I was not too surprised to find spirituality virtually prohibited and banished from the academic discipline that claims to be the scientific study of suicide. But I was surprised – indeed stunned and appalled – to see that the first-person voice of suicidal people was also almost totally absent. This was made all the more stark by the strong presence within suicidology of those bereaved by suicide, which is another important – but very different – first-person voice on the experience of suicide.

My investigations led me to conclude that there are several reasons why the first-person voice of suicidal people is largely absent from suicidology. None of them are good. I'll mention just a couple. First, many experts hold the view that people who survive a suicide attempt can tell us little, if anything, about those who succeed in killing themselves. Some pedantically argue that suicide by definition requires a dead body, so survivors, such as me, cannot tell us anything useful about successful or 'real' suicide attempts. This attitude represents a slightly sanitised version of the common prejudice that the only genuine suicide attempt is a successful one. This is not only offensive to people like me, it is also contradicted by the hard quantitative data so loved by these very same experts, which show that most suicides are preceded by at least one unsuccessful attempt.

But the main reason, I believe, why suicidology pays so little attention to the suicidal person is that suicide is considered irrational madness, so, almost by definition, such people are seen to have nothing useful to contribute to the rational, scientific study of suicide. This is just one of numerous examples of how suicidology uses its scientific pretensions to exclude not only the spiritual and the subjective but also anything that it deems to be irrational. I think this also suits many suicidologists very nicely because many of them really do not want to have any real contact with actual suicidal people.

Dissenting voices within suicidology

I must mention a couple of notable exceptions within mainstream suicidology who do give genuine attention to the actual suicidal person. The first is Professor Edwin S Shneidman, a pioneer in the field who was the founder and inaugural President of the American Association of Suicidology in the early 1960s. Shneidman put the suicidal person at the centre of his study of suicide, saying that:

> *... the keys to understanding suicide are made of plain language...*
> *the ordinary everyday words that are found in the verbatim reports of*
> *beleaguered suicidal minds (1996: viii).*

He then coined the term *psychache*, which he defined as psychological pain due to thwarted or distorted psychological needs, as the basis for his central idea that 'every case of suicide stems from excessive psychache'. Psychache is conceptually very different to the (notional) medical illness of depression, which Shneidman saw as the dominant but unhelpful influence in suicidology in recent decades:

> *No branch of knowledge can be more precise than its intrinsic subject*
> *matter will allow. I believe that we should eschew specious accuracy. I*
> *know that the current fetish is to have the appearance of precision – and*
> *the kudos and vast monies that often go with it – but that is not my*
> *style. Nowadays, the gambit used to make a field appear scientific is to*
> *redefine what is being discussed. The most flagrant current example is to*
> *convert the study of suicide, almost by sleight of hand, into a discussion*
> *of depression – two very different things (2002: 200).*

Sadly Professor Shneidman died in 2009, age 91, lamenting the current medical dominance of the academic discipline that he helped to establish. Fortunately there are a few dissenting voices within modern suicidology that carry his legacy forward. In particular, the Aeschi Group, named after the Swiss village where they meet every two years, is a group of eminent suicidologists who challenge the dominant discourse in suicidology today.[1] Like Shneidman, they put the suicidal person at the centre of their study of suicide and regard what we say about our suicidal feelings – in our own words – as the 'gold standard' for understanding suicide. I regard the Aeschi Group as the *only* innovative, critical and creative voice within mainstream suicidology today.

---

1. See www.aeschiconference.unibe.ch

Suicidology is part of the problem

By the time I completed my PhD I was convinced that suicidology is part of the problem rather than the solution in our efforts to prevent suicide. Let me say this again in rather stronger language – suicidology currently contributes to, rather than reduces, the suicide toll. In order to justify this serious accusation, I now want to look at the two biggest obstacles I see in suicide prevention. This will take our story here beyond academic suicidology into the politics of suicide, but we must keep in mind that suicidology occupies a critical role in this politics.

Suicidology is part of the problem – stigma

The first major obstacle to suicide prevention is typically called stigma, though it should be called by its correct name, discrimination, which immediately takes us into the political realm. Suicidology, along with the wider suicide prevention industry, regularly highlights stigma as a central issue, but at the same time fails to see the stigmatising effects of its own attitudes and practices. A couple of examples of this have already been mentioned, but there are plenty of others, in particular the pathologising and medical labelling of suicidal people.

But what typically fails to get mentioned in the discussion of stigma is that its major source are the mental health laws that make second-class citizens of suicidal people. These laws not only discriminate against and stigmatise the suicidal individual, they are also the legal foundation of mental health systems based on depriving people of their liberty and then forcing unwanted medical treatment on them. Suicidal people, like everybody else, do not want to lose their liberty and be assaulted by medical violence, so we find that mental health services are being deliberately avoided by the very people they are supposed to help. At the very least, this contributes to the suicide toll by failing those in need of help with their suicidal feelings. But even worse, some suicidal people who do make contact with mental health services are finally pushed over the edge into suicide by the violence they encounter from these services. And even worse again, detention and medical violence can actually trigger suicidal feelings in people who have never previously been suicidal.

For some years I have been asking the suicide and other mental health experts in Australia whether our mental health laws help or hinder suicide prevention. In particular, I ask them for any evidence that detention and forced treatment actually helps prevent suicide. There is in fact no scientific evidence for this, for the simple reason that there has been no research into this critically important question. I then point out that if detention and force were to be evaluated by the criteria of medical research, which is not unreasonable given that they are claimed to be life-saving interventions, then the lack of any evidence on either their efficacy or safety would mean that they would simply not be permitted. Despite this, everyone maintains the status quo assumption that force is necessary. But I say it contributes to the suicidal toll, and that, in the absence of proper scientific studies, this is supported by the little evidence that does exist, along with basic human rights principles that violating people's human rights is harmful.

Suicidology's persistent silence on discriminatory, stigmatising and harmful mental health laws represents a tacit acceptance of status quo assumptions that contribute to rather than reduce the suicidal toll. Suicidology is part of the problem of the stigma of suicide.

Suicidology is part of the problem – medicalisation

The second major obstacle to suicide prevention is found at the heart of these mental health laws; it is the medicalisation of suicide. A suicide attempt can have medical consequences, including death, but it is never caused by a medical illness. What causes suicide is a *decision* to kill yourself – a psychological, cognitive decision, not some biological medical terminal illness. It may be that an unbearable medical illness is a factor leading to that decision, but it is not the illness that kills you.

The medicalisation of suicide has arisen alongside the emergence of biological psychiatry as the dominant influence in mental health over the last 30–50 years. A massive global public relations campaign has convinced most people, at least in Western countries like Australia, that most suicides are caused by the medical illness of depression. A recent example in Europe of medical dogma dominating suicide prevention can be seen in a document from the EC-led European Pact for Mental Health and Well-Being (Wahlbeck & Makinen, 2008), which asserts: 'Suicide is primarily an outcome of untreated depressive illness.' Although many people do believe this to be true, many others do not, so it is extraordinary to see a statement like this in a document that claims to be a 'consensus paper'. This belief that suicide is caused by depression has occurred even though the scientific status of depression as a genuine medical illness is hotly contested. But even if you accept depression as a medical illness, it is not a terminal illness. Depression does not *cause* suicide. The most that can be said is that there appears to be some correlation between depression and suicide, but it is a serious mistake to confuse correlation with causation.

More realistically, though, the medical label of depression represents nothing more than an indication of emotional distress, which may be due to a wide range of causes – physical (biological), mental (psychological), relational (social/cultural) and/or spiritual. Blaming suicide on the notional medical illness of depression leads to some dangerous consequences, such as the misguided view that suicide can be prevented by medical treatment, in particular by treatment with antidepressants. It is time that the massive antidepressant experiment of the last 20–30 years is declared a failure, at least for suicide prevention. Another harmful consequence is that we now know that psychiatric labelling stigmatises – rather than destigmatises, as was hoped – those of us who experience extreme emotional distress or other disturbing states of consciousness (Pescosolido et al, 2010). But the most serious consequence of blaming suicide on the medical illness of depression is that, if we believe that depression causes suicide, then we fail to look for the real underlying reasons why a person chooses to die rather than to live.

Suicidology's embrace of depression as the primary causal explanation of suicide does not come from any good science and is demonstrably due to medical ideological dogma. Driven by fear and ignorance and prejudice, society continues to panic in response to suicide and seeks to contain and control suicidal people. The state then calls on the medical profession as a willing accomplice to provide a justification for the use of force under the guise of medical treatment. A little scrutiny reveals that this is not based on science or any rational argument but rather on ideological dogma. Suicidology is part of the problem, rather than the solution, in our efforts to prevent suicide.

Alternatives to (medicalised) suicidology

Looking for alternatives to suicidology's current thinking about suicide, the first step is to reconceptualise how we think about suicide. We can begin by reinvigorating Shneidman's concept of psychache, but I think we can take it even further.

Suicide as a crisis of the self

Suicide is best understood as a *crisis of the self*, rather than the consequence of some notional mental illness. I say this for several reasons. First of all, the self is the 'sui' in suicide, and both the victim and the perpetrator of any suicidal act. It should be the most important concept in the study of suicide, but suicidology gives it remarkably little attention.

Second, thinking about suicide as a crisis of the self is much closer to what it feels like to live with suicidal feelings. The starting point for the study of suicide should be what suicidal feelings mean to those who live them – the first-person knowledge of those who know suicidal feelings 'from the inside'.

Third, any reasonable concept of the self will automatically be a more holistic approach than the current shallow medical approach that reduces us all to biochemical robots. Our sense of self encompasses not only our physical, biological being but also the mental, social, cultural, historical and spiritual aspects of our being.

Thinking about suicide as a crisis of the self also goes a long way towards breaking the stigma of suicide. We all have our own personal sense of self. We have all had times when our sense of self has felt challenged, wounded or in crisis in some way or other. This may not necessarily have been a suicidal crisis but the experience and knowledge of a self in crisis is something that we all share and are familiar with. This automatically breaks down the 'them-and-us' thinking that lies behind much of the stigma around suicide, so that there is no longer a them-and-us, only us.

'Mentally healthy' communities

Another conclusion from my research is that real progress in reducing the suicide toll will not come through interventions with actively suicidal people. These interventions are important for those individuals, and I'll say more about this soon, but I doubt that this approach will yield really significant reductions in the overall numbers. Rather, the key to suicide prevention is to create communities where people are less likely to get suicidal in the first place.

Another way of saying this is that the key to suicide prevention is 'mentally healthy' communities. I don't particularly like this language but most people get the idea of what's meant by it. When I ask myself what a mentally healthy community would actually look like, I struggle because it is such a huge question and one that we really should be asking more frequently. It also makes me acutely aware that the society I live in is very obviously not a mentally healthy one.

But one thing I'm certain of is that a mentally healthy community would be capable of having a sensible conversation about suicide. And again, that this is currently not the case for the society I live in.

Talking about suicide

So the most important thing we can do to reduce the suicide toll is to open up a broad, ongoing community conversation about suicide. This is not only to help prevent suicidal feelings from arising in the first place but also to help those who are actively suicidal. This conversation is essential to bring suicide out of the closet as a public health issue and to dismantle the toxic taboo around it – to break the poisonous silence that feeds the fears, ignorance and prejudices about suicide.

This conversation is also necessary to reclaim this issue as a public issue that is not owned by the professional experts who have failed us so badly. We need to reclaim our personal power, both individually and collectively, and take ownership and responsibility for suicide prevention. This also is about our sense of self – this time our collective rather than individual sense of self: the 'we' rather than the 'I'; the first-person plural as distinct from the first-person singular.

When I then ponder what this conversation might look like, there are a couple of key elements that must be a part of it. First of all, suicidal people themselves must be at the very centre of this conversation. This can be challenging and perhaps too hard for some people who are currently actively suicidal, so great care is required. But there are many thousands of survivors of suicide attempts who are able to speak of their suicidal experiences. This conversation must embrace and engage with this vast untapped wealth of knowledge and expertise on what it means to be suicidal.

I have been calling for this community conversation on suicide for many years. But only recently did I realise that this conversation is not just about breaking the taboo around suicide and exploring more useful ways of preventing suicide. It finally dawned on me that this conversation is its own suicide prevention strategy or intervention – that talking sensibly about suicide can prevent suicide.

Imagine a person, perhaps a young person struggling with their sense of self, who begins to doubt whether they want to continue living. Imagine that this person lives in a community where they know they can talk about these feelings safely – a mentally healthy community. Imagine a community where there are safe spaces where this person can take some time out to consider the big questions that are arising for them. Imagine, if you can, a community where suicidal feelings are respected rather than feared and despised, and where the suicidal person is welcomed rather than shunned. I find it difficult to imagine this community. But I can dream.

A radical challenge

I'll finish with what I've been surprised to learn is in fact the most radical alternative, the most radical challenge, that I can make about how we think about suicide. At the very beginning of the book from my PhD, *Thinking about Suicide*, I speak directly to my fellow suicidal soulmates and invite them 'to honour and respect your suicidal feelings as real, legitimate and important' (2010).

When I wrote this I didn't think it was such a big statement but the feedback I've had from fellow survivors has shown me that this is perhaps the most important thing I say in the whole book. One illustration of this is the response of a friend and fellow survivor in Melbourne, who kindly allowed me to use her words on the back cover of the book:

I have never before read anything relating to suicide that speaks of suicidal feelings as being worthy of respect. The possibility that I may actually be able to honour these feelings is a totally new concept, one which has proven to be a catalyst for change and personal growth.

A rose garden for suicide prevention

Most of the key elements of my rose garden vision for suicide prevention seem rather obvious to me, but they need to be stated because many of them fly in the face of the current thinking and practices of mainstream suicidology.

1. **Prohibit psychiatric violence – stop beating us up**
   Legally sanctioned psychiatric force is the primary source of the stigma against suicide and suicidal people. It also does not work as a suicide prevention strategy. On the contrary, psychiatric violence can make a suicidal crisis more severe and can even trigger suicidal feelings in someone who has previously never been suicidal. Real progress with suicide prevention cannot commence until the current reliance on psychiatric force is abolished.

2. **Demedicalise suicide**
   The second major obstacle to progress with suicide prevention is the inappropriate and excessive medicalisation of suicide. Suicide prevention requires a whole-of-person, whole-of-community, holistic approach, which is not well served by the current medical dominance of suicidology and suicide prevention.

3. **Rethinking suicide as a crisis of the self**
   Hand in hand with the demedicalising of suicide must come a rethinking of suicide in non-medical terms. The concept of psychache is useful here, but thinking about suicide as a crisis of the self is also proposed.

4. **Mentally healthy communities**
   The purpose of mental health policies and programmes needs to shift away from the treatment of mental illness (including so-called prevention

and early intervention strategies based on the medical model) to a model based on the promotion of psychosocial wellbeing. The aim here is to create communities where suicidal feelings, and other forms of psychosocial distress, are much less likely to arise in the first place. It will also create communities that are much more able to respond constructively to such crises if and when they do arise.

5. **Safe spaces for suicidal people**
    Perhaps the most critical component of a mentally healthy community is to have safe spaces for people who are feeling suicidal (or other forms of psychosocial distress). These can be simply for a period away from life's daily demands in order to spend some time with these feelings in a safe and supportive environment. But they can also be spaces where stories of crisis and distress can be told and shared, which in turn can often then be the starting point for genuine healing.

6. **Social model of madness**
    The medical model of suicide – and of all forms of psychosocial distress – is a demonstrable failure that frequently causes great harm, including deaths by suicide, and urgently needs to be replaced. Our disability cousins have long recognised this failure of the medical model and have developed a social model of disability that is now enshrined in the UN Convention on the Rights of Persons with Disabilities (CRPD). This social model, and the CRPD, can form the basis for the radical redesign and rebuilding of mental health systems that will promote rather than diminish psychosocial wellbeing and 'mentally healthy' communities.

7. **Survivors as researchers**
    As a psychiatric survivor who has been fortunate enough to have done a PhD on my particular topic of suicide, I make the (simple) point that a vital key to bringing more of the survivor perspective into research is to have more survivors as researchers. It follows from this that there needs to be affirmative action programmes, such as scholarships, to make this happen.

8. **Funding – stop wasting money on what we know does not work**
    We must stop wasting (lots of) money on what we already know does not work. And this reminds us of the political struggle we face before we will see the radical transformation of our mental health systems that is so urgently needed.

References

Burgess P, Pirkis J, Jolley D, Whiteford H, Saxena S (2004). Do nations' mental health policies, programs and legislation influence their suicide rates? An ecological study of 100 countries. *Australian and New Zealand Journal of Psychiatry 38*(11-12): 933-999.

Churchill R, Owen G, Singh S, Hoptoff M (2007). *International Experiences of Using Community Treatment Orders.* London: Department of Health/Institute of Psychiatry.

Michel K, Jobes D (eds) (2010). *Building a Therapeutic Alliance with the Suicidal Patient.* Washington DC: American Psychological Association Press.

Kisely SR, Campbell LA (2014). Compulsory community and involuntary outpatient treatment for people with severe mental disorders. *Cochrane Database of Systematic Reviews 12*: Art. No. CD004408. DOI: 10.1002/14651858.CD004408.pub4

Pescosolido B, Martin J, Long S, Medina T, Phelan J, Link B (2010). 'A disease like any other'? A decade of change in public reactions to schizophrenia, depression, and alcohol dependence. *American Journal of Psychiatry 167*(11): 1321–1330.

Shneidman ES (1996). *The Suicidal Mind.* Oxford: Oxford University Press.

Shneidman ES (2002). *Comprehending Suicide: landmarks in 20th century suicidology.* Washington DC: American Psychological Association.

Webb D (2010). *Thinking about Suicide: contemplating and comprehending the urge to die.* Ross-on-Wye: PCCS Books.

Wahlbeck K, Mäkinen M (eds) (2008). *Prevention of Depression and Suicide.* Consensus paper. Luxembourg: European Communities.

11

Community Treatment Orders: once a rosy deinstitutional notion?

Erick Fabris

Community Treatment Orders (CTOs) have been touted as an alternative to extended or repeated hospitalisations. They have even been considered as a tool for recovery (St. Joseph's, 2015). This is instructive for anyone attempting to create alternatives to psychiatry, especially as we begin to consider a political practice beyond therapies. The lesson is not only a matter of how our practices can be co-opted or mass-produced, but also how we represent and practise our 'alternatives'. My feeling is that we are stuck in the old dichotomy between force and freedom, much debated in Western help professions, even as the professions create ever-new forms for transcending this dichotomy. However our resistance – first our claim to autonomy, then our development of democratic or mutual aid, and later non-didactic collectives – provides us with examples of practices that do not impose first and offer choices later. In this sense, we may not be able to theorise the correct alternative, the rose garden itself, but we may develop some ways of avoiding practices like compulsory treatment and all it brings.

CTOs and other forms of off-site civil commitment (involuntary outpatient committal, extended leave agreements etc) parody the 'right to choose' as a way of excusing their inherent compulsoriness. As such, they may seem to some like a form of deinstitutionalisation. As long as we ignore the 'order' and concentrate on the 'community', we will be spellbound. We can live and learn, love and work off-site, all from the comfort of what we call home. As long as we ignore the tranquilliser in the medicine, or at least how many of us have to be tied down to be medicated before we say yes to psychiatry and no to 'withdrawal', CTOs fulfil the system's hope of a treatment that doesn't seem like treatment at all. Imagine a blameless treatment. Imagine if tranquillisers or electroshock were not the primary modes of treatment, and psychiatry found a cleaner, more socially conscious methodology. Here is the pitfall: the therapeutic project itself. If we resist the drive to therapy, the urge to treat, we may avoid psychiatry's embrace, and its ghosts.

Is mutual aid free from coercion? Probably not, but at least it's not brandishing statutory compulsion as its calling card. Some might say that anything done mutually escapes coercive practices. Perhaps psychiatrists and psychologists from oppressed groups should be considered survivors of broader systems and therefore natural allies, their coercive practices merely a fault of the founders of those professions? From the opposite position, in which individual responsibility is independent of structure, it would be impossible for me to pretend that a writer is not also a part of such systems. Any meaning can be twisted back on itself; any intent may be suspect, or inscrutable (except to psychoanalysis, perhaps, or some other mystic presence). However, we might at least question the drive to therapy as already embedded in the bulwark of pathologising and its asocial projections.

Can we ever win?

'Winning', as Charlie Sheen might admit, is not always so easy. George Clooney did it well at the Golden Globes in 2015 when he said he was humbled to find his love fulfilled his dreams. I assume he meant marriage to Amal Alamuddin did not tear him away from political activism but reinforced it, because she was already working in a field towards which Clooney could only aspire. The privilege to serve from a position of power is related, though distinct from, the power to change, facilitate or support one another. In this way, the perfect treatment may not be treatment at all.

Though I was humbled, in one sense, by drugging and locked hospitalisation, I felt a different humility when an academic press was willing to publish a psychiatric survivor protest like mine (Fabris, 2011). My book, *Tranquil Prisons*, published by the University of Toronto Press, was a shoring up of whatever I learned from 20 years of activism – some of it good, some of it bad – and it was a major labour of love. I'm glad it is doing well, and I would not be writing this if I hadn't tried writing academically, but something about its conclusion has stuck with me. Psychiatric appropriation of survivor work continues relentlessly. After years of struggling to be heard, it seemed incredible that I might be one of the first, privileged people to make survivor protests 'visible' to academics who have the power to contest power. But, after a few years of academising my protest, theorising my identities and reconsidering my practices, I feel less optimistic.

The division between overtly 'psych' (ie. psychiatric, psychological, psychotherapeutic, psychoanalytic...) and unabashedly anti-professional is only one of the intersectional lenses to be addressed when we theorise the perfect rose garden. As a white, heterosexual, able-bodied, cisgender, male body travelling through academia, I took up identity labour/politics as a prerequisite to theorising my own resistance to psych oppression. I wonder if I have done a disservice to a form of resistance that is still unrecognised among mainstreaming, sanesplaining moral movements. I pretend it hardly matters when madness is constructed as incomprehensible. Yet moral superiority, which depends on intellectual superiority, is the kind of mentalism that flies under the radar of anti-oppression. If there is an alternative to psychiatry, it may come at the price of being incomprehensible to mainstreaming, saner movements, including medical model user/consumer activisms.

Thus how we 'socialise' around disaffection, distress, disease and all manner of otherness in sanist society is tied to how we 'imagine' divergence of thought as a matter of 'solidarity'. I can't write these words without acknowledging that they are loaded, because pushing for 'alternatives' begs the question, 'Alternative to what?' – how was it once alternative, how is it now the same and, finally, how do we feel about changing it? How are the alternatives already framed in the demands and aims of the system that tries to fix us? If the industry of coercive care tends to steal activists' ideas, what should we do to address this?

Writing as resistance

Let's consider writing as a form of protest that can easily be usurped by systems seeking 'newness'. The privilege of writing worries me. It's a bit like being the first student to put their hand up in class. The teacher benefits from this enthusiasm. Meanwhile other students must continue to demonstrate learning from the lesson. We who were 'smart in school' were rewarded in ways that made common knowledge seem 'normal'. Writing is the ability to normalise feelings and ideas and make them consistent with common sense, and thus supports the experiences and thought already inscribed. For example, what happens if I try to overexpose the project of mentalism and sanism? I could rally and promote and correct and inform. Do I not then conform to the anti-oppression politics that missed these ideas in the first place?

In my experience, the act of writing and editing glories in understandability. Like having an emotion massaged into the background of awareness, working a text to comprehensibility reflects the search for prowess in psychiatric society. We who are grammatical and intelligible escape the fray. But there are consequences to massaging out every bump in a piece of writing. Bumps add textures that make expression identifiable and compelling. Clear writing is good for signs, recipes, and instruction manuals, but it's not enough for works of the heart. Academic presses may imagine the universal audience ready for anything, if we're just 'clear' enough. But maybe a lot of people are not willing to commit to academic prose precisely because it is so managed. Even style manuals admit the rules do not guarantee good writing. I have met several people who've tried complex or confounding prose, and if it works they keep reading. Shakespeare is a case in point.

There are second language learners like me whose usages are simpler or lack subtlety. I learned English in my youth and now am relearning Italian slowly. *Non parlo bene l'italiano ma provo ancora* (*I don't speak Italian well but I'm still trying* – I'm almost sure that's *not* how an Italian would say it). We benefit from the occasional simple sentence in a news article or from the least difficult style in a collection. But we struggle on with the more involved sentences or articles, knowing that we won't achieve a fully nuanced understanding of a culture in just a few readings. I read to be exposed to a new way of understanding and thinking, not simply to master it in a day. And this speaks to the question of understandability: sense is sometimes nonsense, and good writing is sometimes bad.

But more germane to this project, the problem of psychiatry demanding understandability from its wards makes any demand on survivors for readable prose a bit onerous. It would be like asking a refugee to dress more 'respectably' before coming to a hearing on some matter. It's our right to express ourselves as we do; we didn't get here without a struggle. We need to read that struggle in our work. It's not that every survivor who's been silenced writes like any other, or that our lost emotions are a new language. It's that we deserve to be considered, bumps, bruises and all. To tell us how to testify is like telling an outsider to check their accent first; it's a denial of lived experience. Often this argument is mistaken for a *Sturm und Drang* romanticism, as is anything opposing drug management in mental health care. But it's just about the right to write as we need. Does that even make sense?

Along with this writing privilege and the privileges of maleness, whiteness, ablebodiedness, anglophony, and a host of other normalcies, I should not neglect to mention 'capable-mindedness' and 'voluntariness' under psychiatric care and control as models of sound societies. These two terms show privileges yet to be theorised in the identarian academy. The sanist society is indeed a place where the most 'sound' of us excel, while the less understood lag behind, get into trouble, get held back and get lost. How do I exploit or appropriate their future writing by theorising oppression? And yet not writing doesn't solve the problem either.

I recently had a taste of losing this privilege of making meaning, or representing oneself. I was in Italy last summer, doing organic farming work and learning a bit about my own cultural background, but I didn't speak much Italian. It was interesting being ignored and condescended to, sometimes out of pity rather than malice, much as when I was looked down upon for being a mental patient, and when I was first learning English as a boy. Even 'new' Italians would skip my attempts at communication in order to get things done. I was an outsider in my own culture.

It was in Italy that I realised Italian culture was itself too complex for me to understand. It was as messy as my Canadian settler technosociety – indeed, more messy. It was ancient, and it was saturated with cultures from all over, while at the same time presenting a singular nationalism that couldn't be mistaken for any other European nation. It spoke to my understanding of how groupthink, which is the basis for sanity or any 'agreement' about reality, goes deeper than ethnicity or even family, insofar as these are constructions rather than essences. Ironies in identity reveal the complexities of the art of knowing and doing: the mad movement becomes the Mad movement, and in that shift it mirrors itself, in one person, maybe in many.

Knowing the right way is also an act of confusion and desperation (madness is normalcy and vice versa). I came away from Italy feeling very unsettled, as if my privilege was only skin deep, and under it were layers of other privileges (and losses) I'd never before considered. With my English-North American globetrotting on one hand and my Italian-Vatican centre of the universe on the other, I didn't think about how I was suffering in a way that could not be named. It may be mentalism, or sanism, I don't know. But this unspoken experience speaks to the problem of alternatives, and how the promise of knowing another's way is always fraught with complexity at many levels.

Fighting for control

Mad politics runs the gamut from medical to social models and beyond, from fantasists to post-humanists and more, and in this 'sense' mad politics is like race, gender or class politics in their diversity. But it's also unlike sanestream politics, in the sense that Mad movements are always first 'non-sense' (somewhat like any other movement, but not exactly like any other movement), and this is not as magical or wondrous as we could have hoped. This unintelligibility may be a gift in disguise for anyone who wants to imagine 'imagining' anew. But in the intelligible world, we've seen people push for more psychiatrists based on their own 'experiential knowledge' and otherwise we've seen people break into academic publishing by fighting psychiatrisation, as I tried to do. To what end do we work for change?

In my book, I took to task the idea of 'assertive community treatment' whose endgame was 'Community Treatment Orders', and tried to theorise its beginnings and ends. Was such treatment not an industrial solution to the deinstitutionalisation debates of the 1960s – a good idea turned into a commercial success? And what was its purpose other than selling drugs, drugging, and the concept of the chemical life? As many have said, one goal of compulsory care outside the ward was to bring institutionalisation into the 'community'. What I argue in *Tranquil Prisons* is that it also tries to bring incarceration into the body through psychopharmacy. But in relation to alternative care, treatment orders show us how a good idea goes big and possibly bad, and how alternatives like medicalising madness in the 1800s are adapted for power. Not all good ideas spoil, however, and we need to think about how to keep fresh ideas fresh.

One of our best ideas has been to socialise with one another. I think we need to rediscover and rediscover ways to 'socialise' out of psych control. In this sense, the rose garden that we aren't promised is not just 'social', or 'open' (in the sense of transparent and accountable); it's not simply some better care option on the state's menu; it is always there, being questioned and reconsidered. This constant re-questioning is necessary to re-inventing practices. More importantly, it's necessary to our understanding of mutuality. Questioning, which seems to run away with us in theorising, might actually ground us in 'practice', where we balk at the notion of 'reinventing the wheel'. I think of gears, rollers and castors, and I wonder if re-invention is a better way to consider multiple ways of theorising, politicising and resisting.

Likewise, direct protest demanding an end to force may look and feel active, but ultimately the state is unlikely to introduce a more caring system of support simply because it's less expensive and healthier. It will leave that to volunteers like us and merely soften the torture, as the UN calls compulsory care. As you probably have heard, the UN Convention on the Rights of Persons with Disabilities (United Nations, 2007) pushes for governments to abandon imposing treatments on people with disabilities, including psychosocial disabilities. Could it be that, in order to understand how change occurs in any system, we need to allow for people to opt out of reform?

CTOs are a prime example of how not to end psychiatry. A substitute for incarceration merely changes the method of control. As I've argued, people can be restrained internally, through the body, as much as by external constraints or environmental barriers. In that sense, not only do CTOs recreate incarceration, they use iatrogenic reactions including 'suicidality' as a rationale for further control. The body is first conceived as 'ill' or 'mad' and, as it is made sick with drugs, it can always be blamed for the failure of the intervention and the need for improved (or more intensive) interventions. This is what I call a 'cycling of chemistry' in *Tranquil Prisons* – a sort of 'pre-blame the victim' approach to institutionalisation. It normalises abuse, iatrogenesis and narrative control of the victim.

Delusions of alterity

So, again, one of the problems with devising alternatives is that of trying to fix bad ideas. Are we deluded in trying? But delusion is a dishonest word – one the state likes to use as a rationale for imposing care. When such care is completely confused, as it is when a control-based economy attempts to 'care', there is no way we can hope for reasonable discussion. The term is already unreasonable or meaningless, and we need to avoid recycling that mistaken superiority, that sanism. There is no sanity except what we individually take to be real, especially when what is assumed to be reality requires that we coerce people into treatment for their bad ideas and behaviours in a violent world, or that we debate whether coercion in fact 'works' in a clinical sense by reducing 'delusions' and 'oppositionality' in patients. We dare not abandon making sense in a sanist society, but should we therefore refuse to make nonsense in any way?

I believe there is no way to prevent the investors and their machines from using the next best hope as part of their marketing strategy. Which is why I say we must keep trying to avoid a falling back to 'least restrictive' options. We need to keep moving forward, towards doing something mutual, not by formula, but not by accident either. This would require constant change. While bankers frequently change their tactics, they seldom change their opposition to our hiding our money under a mattress. The word 'mutual' itself is easily appropriated, and some of our mutual ways could be too, but mutuality is not a hiding place; mutuality is our version of the bank.

To participate in the preservation, rather than become moguls in it, is important to divest from expertise and the next best therapy. We can't play the role of disinterested helper or saviour, which is of course what the condescending worker does. Is it ever possible for us to ask for something for ourselves, and so become 'included' ourselves, as a part of the change we want in the world? In this sense the CTO as a mode of 'care' that encourages us to stay compliant with medical expertise is a lesson for reformers and abolitionists of psychiatry.

'So how did it feel to go crazy?' someone might ask you over brunch. The temptation is to keep calm and carry on: 'Well, you know, it was a bit like, "What's the weirdest thing you've done...?"'. Of course, you can't explain in 'normal' language what it means to see the world utterly differently... not just in terms of 'belief' or 'worldview' but as a body with completely altered organs and senses, and as a heart with completely open gates and windows. The response could be, 'I hate it when people ask me that!' But that unforgiving answer belies a smarter-than-thou attitude. I still believe that anger directed at individuals for their adaptation to oppressive influences ('ignorance') is a self-destructive urge played out within groups. The group that polices ignorance refuses to learn from its own ignorance.

Rather than go out into the world telling people at every turn when they are sanist in a sanist world, I would rather offer time to allow people to discover for themselves what it is to be seen as mad, mislabelled, have treatment forced on you, and be mentally incapacitated. Time and open questions might change a culture of coercion to a culture of relating, even between ignorances. And so the idea of socialising out of psychiatric control-care includes the idea of not marketing it, not sanesplaining it, not boxing it for the factory floor. This brings with it the attendant problem that it might not even be recognisable to many people as anything like an alternative.

Concluding?

The conundrum of how we change dominant systems without risking dominance is something I find quite discomforting. While we say we will fight to change society and make it more accommodating and less controlling, the idea of fighting itself is wide open to exploitation and redirection into the next 'new boss, same as the old boss'. In Italy I was planting and harvesting on organic gardens, and saw for the first time artichoke plants with their beautiful purple flowers, but often my activities were performed to meet the demands of the marketplace. To cultivate roses may not be what the Mad movements need, and to promise roses would be psychiatric.

There are several social movements that pushed for something more than simple truths, including the Jungian and Laingian schools. Although these professionals had life experiences that sound 'mad' and although they have largely been ignored by biological 'care', their answers to the questions they faced may be instructive as well. But rather than follow them into their answers, we might reinvent their questions altogether. Why not ask ourselves how we can find ways of being with one another without hurting one another or rebranding coercion and force? Why not see life not as therapeutic or 'crazy' but rather as always different and always differently so?

I think, with these starting points, our ideas about how to move to less coercive ways, even 'systems' of interaction, cannot be packaged; they are perpetual beginnings. How do we live with change so that we are fair to one another and ourselves? Is this too much to ask? I have not been able to keep my thinking and my questions changing, like life, and my life has made me far from perfect. However I feel that striving for a dynamic, changeable way of being is teaching me to look outside the garden.

References

Fabris E (2011). *Tranquil Prisons: chemical incarceration under community treatment orders*. Toronto, Canada: University of Toronto Press.

St. Joseph's Healthcare (2015). *Community Treatment Order Program (CTO)*. [Online.] Hamilton, ON: St Joseph's Heathcare. www.stjoes.ca/health-services/mental-health-addiction-services/mental-health-services/schizophrenia-and-community-integration-service-scis-/community-treatment-order-program-cto- (accessed 3 April, 2015).

United Nations (2007). *Convention on the Rights of Persons with Disabilities*. A/RES/61/106. New York: United Nations. http://www.un.org/disabilities/convention/conventionfull.shtml (accessed 3 April, 2015).

SURVIVOR-CONTROLLED PRACTICE

12

Becoming part of each other's narratives: Intentional Peer Support

Shery Mead and Beth Filson

Since the 1990s people who identify as having some type of extreme experience have been hired in the publicly funded mental health system in the US to provide peer support services. Peer support was introduced without any substantial change to the policies and procedures that would support mutual, reciprocal relationships. Over time many peer supporters have adapted to the existing system with peer support looking more and more like clinical support. The inequality of one-way helping relationships has become the norm. This chapter will explore Intentional Peer Support (IPS),[1] which offers another view of mutuality. In IPS, mutuality is understood as a practice of dialogue where both people attempt to understand their experiences of power and powerlessness.

What is Intentional Peer Support?

Intentional Peer Support is a process of relationship that seeks to explore the events in our lives and the stories we create out of them. Through dialogue, new meaning evolves as we compare and contrast how we have come to know what we know. Our shared stories create communities of intentional healing and hope. IPS challenges the notion that people need to leave their communities for specialised treatment. When people share their stories without others imposing meanings on them, this creates social change.

---

1. You can find out more about Intentional Peer Support at: www.intentionalpeersupport.org

A brief history of Intentional Peer Support

Intentional Peer Support grew out of survivor/researcher/writer Shery Mead's work with women who had experienced domestic abuse. Through their time together, Shery became aware that people live out of many different stories. For example, the stories Shery heard when women were talking to her about the abuses or even when they 'played' their experiences in her trauma survivors music group were very different from the stories the same women told once they had been involved with the mental health system. They went from talking about themselves as strong, resilient survivors to referring to themselves as 'mentally ill'.

Shery decided to find some way to work with the idea that stories about who we are can be redefined. She saw herself in the women around her – others who had become stuck in a mental illness story that was not of their own choosing or making. She wanted to find out whether, through dialogue, they might be able to redefine themselves and the meaning of their experiences.

In 1995 Shery started Stepping Stones, a peer-run crisis alternative to psychiatric hospitalisation in New Hampshire. Stepping Stones was the first totally peer-run respite house; people who came there did not fear hospitalisation if or when they talked about intense feelings, including when they wanted to die. Rather than assessing each other, participants and staff were free to discover their connections with each other. This ability to sit with discomfort, rather than respond to it with fear, led to deep connection among community members.

They started new groups and organised new approaches as old stories were re-examined and new stories were tried out. Through this process they discovered they were interacting differently. They no longer talked about their various diagnoses or disability checks; rather, they communicated through the lens of strengths and possibilities. The story of disability was no longer useful. As they continued to play with new assumptions and new beliefs, each person wrote new realities.

The three principles of Intentional Peer Support

Intentional Peer Support relationships are guided by three principles and four tasks.

First principle: learning about rather than problem solving

What gets called 'mutuality' is often based in subtle power differences between the helper and the person being helped: when the focus is on me helping you, no matter how much I talk about mutuality and equality, it is always going to be my agenda pushing you. Even when I say, 'I'm here to help you figure out what you want,' there is a subtle power imbalance that maintains disconnection.

For example, how do I know that you do not know what you want? How do I know that what I think is helpful is valuable or even relevant to you? These unexplored questions describe the importance of learning about rather than problem solving or fixing. When the focus is on discovery, the helper's notion of help does not define the nature of the relationship or the story about what is taking place in that relationship – 'She is not working very hard on her goals'; 'He is really committed to recovery'.

Helping relationships all too often dissolve into one-way relationships that may *serve to protect the person who takes on the helper role by excusing him/her from participating in a meaningful way in relationships.*

This gives us some semblance of control. Being in control makes us feel better. This need for comfort and control is often translated into our peer support relationships. When peer support is practised in the mental health system rather than in the community, it intersects with the issues of risk management.

In another example, if I come to you and tell you that I feel like cutting myself, there's a good chance that you will either defer to someone else ('Have you talked to your therapist?') or try to get me to stop feeling that way ('You shouldn't feel like that'). We say these things because it is what has been said to us – it is what we have learned as a result of our contact with the mental health system. Most of us have been taught that risk is unacceptable and that *someone else*, someone who is *trained,* should be responsible for pain.

Intentional Peer Support teaches us that we must 'see' differently if we are to 'get' different results. So what does this 'seeing differently' look like?

Thinking about the first principle, *Learning about rather than problem solving or fixing,* I may want to know more about what cutting means to you. What is the story you have learned about yourself? Has this story been helpful?

If we bring to our relationships the desire to learn about one another, we establish the two-way relationships that are integral to Intentional Peer Support and the principles of mutuality. Dialogue allows us to explore how each of us shapes personal meaning. Learning together takes time; it's about building relationships where new information and new knowledge can emerge. When people are willing to listen to each other's stories without providing analysis, and at the same time compare and contrast experiences, the possibilities for transforming meaning are endless. When we become part of each other's narratives, we not only offer the possibility of alternative and mutually enriching interpretations; our new shared story becomes a way to negotiate future challenges and crises while building community. So if I say to you, 'What is the cutting trying to say?' rather than, 'You should talk to your therapist about that', I may open up a very different story than the one you have learned through your contact with the mental health system.

Second principle: focus on the relationship rather than on the individual

In traditional helping relationships, the focus is on one person, the person being 'helped'. This means only one of us in the relationship is expected to change; only one of us is expected to do something differently. When the focus is on the individual, I may feel like I have done my job only when you make changes based on my perception of the problem. This is a real pitfall for many peers working in organisations where meaning is controlled by the medical system and its inherent roles – for example, the role of the patient or the role of the doctor.

Since community is constructed around mutual regard, one-way relationships, no matter how 'helpful', further isolate the 'patient' – or anyone, for that matter, who is perceived to be less capable of contribution. Through participation in two-way relationships, both parties forge the type of connection that moves them out of their perceived and socially constructed roles (provider and service user/recipient) into the roles of community member. When the focus is on the relationship, rather than on the individual, there is an opportunity to be affected by each other and to know ourselves as integral in the lives of others, and for both people to undergo a process of change as a consequence of the relationship.

So what does this look like in practice? Going back to the example above, we may simply acknowledge that it feels scary when someone says they want to cut and I might also ask you how you would like me to respond when you say you want to cut. Now the focus is on the relationship. It is about both people's needs and, through the dialogue, no one feels coerced or victimised.

Third principle: hope versus fear

Fear is a natural response to anything out of the ordinary. In the realm of mental health, responses to distress are usually based on risk management: ie. I learn that crisis is dangerous and my response is to control and contain that danger.

As we said earlier in this chapter, usually when I react out of fear I do so to make myself more comfortable – and that is often when I take control of the situation. If I am in control or am able to contain whatever feels risky, I am liable to shut down new learning for both of us. If, on the other hand, I believe that something positive will come out of our connection despite my discomfort, then new meaning and new ways of being in the world become possible for both of us.

Returning to our example: let's say you come to me and tell me you feel like cutting. I react out of fear, saying something like, 'Well, I need to take you to the hospital if you feel like that.' Chances are, we'll get right back into a power struggle. Instead, after acknowledging my fear and discomfort, I might say something like, 'What do you hope the cutting will do for you?'

Hope-based responses create a different lens for interpreting what is taking place. They come out of faith that you and I can work through this difficult event, even if we haven't before, by being honest and mutually vulnerable. Hope-based responses create a different lens for interpreting what is and what might be.

The four tasks

We talk about the tasks of Intentional Peer Support as a way of carrying out the principles. There are four tasks, and they do have an order, for reasons we'll explain below.

The first task is *connection* – that place of shared vulnerability where people feel seen and heard. In order to achieve connection, it is useful to validate the other person's experience. In the example above, that could mean just saying to the person who feels like cutting, 'That's such a hard place to be.' We need connection in order to really get to know the other person. Without connection we can easily fall into problem solving, which may drive disconnection. Connection also levels the playing field by getting rid of power differentials that are so often embedded in traditional helping relationships.

The second task is *worldview*. Exploring worldview is about being curious – curious about the other person's perspective, their way of making sense. This is significant because, in order to accomplish this, I have to be aware that my own way of seeing and making sense is simply one truth out of multiple truths. This exploration takes us to a deeper kind of connection, where both of our truths can exist side by side. As we did in learning together rather than problem solving, we might ask what the cutting means or even ask what the cutting is trying to say. You can see why worldview comes after connection: when we ask these types of vulnerable questions without connecting first and sharing in that vulnerability, the person may shut down and even leave.

This takes us to the third task of *mutuality*, which has been a major theme of this chapter. Mutuality is a way of sharing worldviews that doesn't make one person's story more important than the other person's. Mutuality lets me share my way of seeing and understanding what the cutting means. This is often a process of comparing and contrasting our stories in order to make sure we really understand one another. So, using this example, I might say something like, 'I think I can relate. I often go out in my car and scream where no one can hear me. It feels very freeing. Is it like that for you to cut?' Mutuality puts the focus on the relationship rather than on the individual.

The fourth task is *moving towards*. People often start with moving towards in traditional services. We are asked, 'What do you want?' by people wanting to 'empower' us. The trouble with this is that, without first going through connection, then worldview and finally mutuality, we find ourselves responding only on the basis of what we currently know, without insight and without self-awareness. For example, if I asked the person who wanted to cut what she was moving towards without having gone through the other tasks, she might have just said that she didn't want to feel the way she feels any longer. But if I've established a connection with her and asked about her worldview while I am also practising mutuality, she and I may both come to see the cutting as something different. Something new is created beyond what either one of us could have come up with on our own.

These four tasks are a critical component of Intentional Peer Support and really establish it as unique practice, but they are not easy to do. With the mental health system breathing down our backs to achieve 'measurable outcomes', we often fall into old roles with each other.

Challenges

An additional barrier to the kind of change Intentional Peer Support envisions is the fear our society has towards people who are deemed outside of the norm. This fear in turn has infused help with coercion. Risk management – managing or controlling people – has been prioritised over relationships that lead to healing. This further disconnects people from community, strengthening the chasm between *us* and *them*.

Peer support has become many things to many people. From sharing personal stories, to becoming 'role models', to giving advice based on lived experience, peer support has more often than not ended up looking like clinical support. The inequality of one-way helping relationships has become the norm.

By default, mental health organisations contradict the principles of Intentional Peer Support through the following:

- mandatory reporting
- policies regarding diagnosis and treatment
- contractual/funding constraints around who I can see
- agreements about how long we can have a relationship for
- policies directing boundaries around peer relationships.

The possibilities

The potential for Intentional Peer Support lies in the assumption that systems and society construct worldviews and these worldviews can change. This is important. Rather than pathologising extreme states, Intentional Peer Support understands them as part of the human experience. This is the meaning of social change – it is bringing into the community the level of empathy usually relegated to professionals. Why is this so important? For one thing, it gets us away from *othering* people and it breaks down many of the assumptions about illness. But it also means that our apparently extreme states are simply normal reactions to dismal events. And when we see normal reactions to dismal events, we find our connections in each other.

The real power of Intentional Peer Support takes place in our conversations and relationships with each other. These conversations can and do occur despite the constraints imposed by the system. They alter the experiential nature of self in relation to others, which in turn begins the process of creating new, more hopeful stories.

Relationships begin with connection. Connection happens when we learn about each other and have opportunities for mutual contribution to the relationship. When one of us is really struggling, we sit with our own discomfort, believing that something good, something that has never happened before, will emerge as a result. We are people responding to our world. When that world becomes dismal, we can unite in communal action because we recognise the social illness, rather than thinking the illness resides in the person.

We believe that the following story provides a snapshot view of this. This event took place in a publicly funded psychiatric hospital.

What people knew of Sam (not his real name) was that he had come to the unit from a forensic hospital and had a history of assaults. For the first week after he arrived he was followed by two psychiatric assistants, who were expected to stay within arm's reach of Sam at all times. On the day this story takes place, Sam had just been released from this close supervision.

Terri and Shay, peer supporters, were half-way through a trauma and recovery group for people on the unit. Sam burst into the room. He'd swiped a mop handle off a cleaning cart out in the hall and he was swinging it around. A member of staff ran behind Sam demanding he hand the mop handle over to him. Sam kept saying he needed it. A rather loud power struggle ensued, with the member of staff demanding the mop handle and Sam insisting that he needed it to help him walk. Tensions quickly mounted as other staff began to congregate in the door to the group room. As is so often the case, it appeared that the only end in sight was going to be a restraint call. But then Terri, one of the peer support group facilitators, welcomed Sam to the group. Sam limped around the table and sat next to her. Shay, the other peer supporter, invited the group members to a different corner of the room to continue their conversation.

As Terri and Sam started talking, staff eventually began backing out of the room.

Terri asked Sam, 'So, what's up with your leg?' Sam looked surprised, then told her he'd hurt it. 'Sorry to hear that,' Terri responded. She asked him how he was getting along. Sam talked about his cane, and how it was helping him.

Sam then asked Terri if he could have some of the food and drink on the table. Terri said that that would be fine, but that she needed something in return – Sam's cane. She explained people seemed to be upset about it. He considered her request. As she prepared a plate for Sam, he handed over the mop handle.

Sam remained with the group as they came back together. They also greeted Sam, and talked about being afraid at first when Sam burst in followed by staff. At one point he intertwined his fingers with Terri's, who acknowledged his 'cool handshake' before turning back to the group. Though Sam did not speak in the group, he listened as members talked about their initial fear over Sam's entrance followed by so many staff, and also what had worked to restore a sense of calm – all the while making sure that Sam was part of the conversation and not being talked about. Members thanked Sam for his willingness to participate and to be with them. They let him know they hoped he would come again. Sam looked perplexed by this 'thank you'. It seemed that this was a first for him: his experience of himself had undergone a radical change from dangerous patient wielding a potential weapon to accepted group member who had something to contribute.

Conclusion

The kinds of conversations created through Intentional Peer Support cannot be separated from the experiences that shape our worldview. This brings *the world* into our conversations, so that we can come together to solve common problems, from inequality and community violence to the issues of our governments or the environment. Intentional Peer Support is about the person in relation to the world and in relation to others. Through relationships – person to his or her world, person to person – what we talk about changes the world.

13

We did it our way: Women's Independent Alcohol Support

Patsy Staddon

Women's Independent Alcohol Support (WIAS) is a small charity run by alcohol survivors and their friends that aims to help other women with alcohol issues find the kind of information and support they need. Service user-controlled academic research (Ettorre, 2007; Staddon, 2009, 2012, 2013, 2014) indicates that this kind of unquestioning and non-judgemental support is often not available in mainstream services, which may in many cases have misunderstood the meaning of the 'presenting issue' of 'alcoholism'.

This is also a difficult area for minority groups in general and for women in particular (Staddon, 2005; Ettorre, 2007; Moon & Staddon, 2015; Serrant, 2015). Shame and lifelong guilt over reneged responsibilities haunt women who have 'failed' to fulfil their prescribed role, in which they are expected to demonstrate femininity and to combine the skills of homemaker and mother, often at the same time as maintaining a paid job. In addition, introducing new ideas about the nature of women's over-drinking, indeed of using alcohol at all, may be viewed negatively by more traditional service user organisations, such as Alcoholics Anonymous, so that working alongside them can be very difficult. Meanwhile, it is increasingly difficult to obtain funding to develop a new non-profit organisation and to support the implementation of new ideas in the field. We hope at WIAS to raise public awareness of the need for alternative services, and to campaign to fund these.

Origins of WIAS

A common understanding of what is commonly understood as alcoholism is that it is an incurable disease, although further physical and mental deterioration may be paused if the person stops drinking alcohol. This understanding holds that people who do stop will still be forever 'in recovery', a state in which they need to be constantly alert to the danger of relapse and, importantly, remain closely networked with organisations such as Alcoholics Anonymous (AA), and attend AA meetings for life. This belief has often been disputed (Hall et al, 2001; Cameron, 1995; Peele, 1995) but remains common both in the alcohol field and in the public domain (Fingarette, 1988; Ettorre, 2007; White, 2008).

One possibility for its too ready acceptance by the medical profession and by lay people may be their distaste and anger when the group that is over-drinking is seen as having less right to be 'out of control'. These groups particularly include mothers and young women, who are seen as icons, respectively, of social responsibility and purity (Ettorre, 2007). Certainly medical frameworks have frequently been shown in research to be riddled with lay prejudice and a culture of blame and misunderstanding (Tidmarsh, Carpenter & Slade, 2003; Vogt, Hall & Marteau, 2006; International Centre for Drug Policy, 2007; Staddon, 2012). Consequently:

> *My identity and my medical condition [may be] seen as inseparable, synonymous, a view still very common in academic journals, taught in medical schools and, unsurprisingly, held by many GPs (Staddon, 2012: 192).*

Sympathy has tended to be reserved for the family and friends of the women concerned. However a woman's alcohol use may have a variety of causes over which she has had minimal or no control. Most common are the issues of domestic abuse (Galvani & Humphreys, 2007) and of mental health problems (Barron, 2004). Additionally, Shaw et al (1999) further identified the role of 'social dissonance' with regard to women's over-drinking. Using substances may express a need to isolate yourself from a society where you feel at a disadvantage and not regarded as of equal value. Unfortunately alcohol services too often fail to consider the difficulties connected with, and compounded by, the struggle to behave and to appear in ways that fit stereotyped ideas of the 'woman's role' (Staddon, 2009).

The WIAS project evolved from service user-controlled academic research that drew attention to these dichotomies of theory and practice. I had recovered from alcoholism, still had mental health problems and neurological impairments, but wanted to challenge the ways that my understanding of myself, and my own concept of recovery, had been dismissed in treatment and in the subsequent 'mutual aid' groups I had attended. I could not accept alcohol addiction as a lifelong condition, whereby you were forever 'in recovery', perpetually vigilant over your need to consume mind-altering substances. This did not match my own developing understanding of why women drink. At the same time my own life was changing: I came out as a woman who loved other women and I needed to see the world through different lenses, as a member of a marginalised group that was proud of its identity. I decided to return to university as a postgraduate student of sociology, particularly to understand how the behaviour expected of women resonated with the politics of power. Where did women's alcohol 'misuse' fit within this syndrome (Staddon, 2012)?

As my research progressed, women with alcohol issues not only replied to my advertisements and magazine, radio and TV requests, but agreed to further in-depth interviews, and to participation in focus groups. Issues such as depression and domestic abuse were the most common triggers to the development of serious alcohol misuse, but mental health problems and poverty were also powerful factors. At the same time alcohol use could be a way of dealing with life, and of facilitating a celebration of the essential self, which was otherwise submerged under the daily routine. Women acknowledged the role of alcohol, whether problematically used or not, in enhancing their pleasure and even their spirituality (Staddon, 2009). The focus groups, originally part of my PhD research, were so successful that they were restarted as support groups after the research, with many other women joining as time went on (Staddon, 2014). These groups continued for over four years in central Bristol.

No blame, no shame – the distinctive WIAS approach

Today, WIAS is a small registered charity. At the time of writing it runs small women's groups within a women's project linked to a probation service, and is about to start similar groups in the community. It hopes soon to be operating a helpline. The purposes of these support services are:

- to help women reflect on their situation without a sense of blame or guilt
- to look at some of the reasons underlying their problems with alcohol use

- to make them aware of other local organisations that might be able to help with specific issues, such as domestic abuse, depression, self-harm, loss of benefits and homelessness.

WIAS is becoming well networked with other third sector organisations, as well as with the statutory services, and aims to be actively supportive, for example in offering introductions to other services, perhaps by accompanying clients to initial interviews.

What makes WIAS different from conventional alcohol 'treatment' organisations is its ethos, its approach and its practice. Alcohol use is understood by WIAS as a normal social activity that, like eating, can easily be taken to extremes and come to take the place of other kinds of nourishment and support. Alternatives that may be less harmful and more helpful are suggested and introduced over time, but the most important central tenet remains unconditional positive regard (Rogers, 1978), whether women are still drinking or not. WIAS has incorporated this understanding in its motto, 'No blame, no shame.' WIAS members are being trained to understand alcohol 'misuse' in this way, whether they facilitate groups, operate the helpline or work as administrators and volunteers.

WIAS sees alcohol problems principally as gendered social issues with multiple causes, each of which may ultimately need to be addressed. Initially women need to speak in confidence on the telephone or in person to another woman who has a supportive and friendly approach and who is able both to listen with compassion and to suggest avenues for finding help as required. Women are likely to need ongoing support in seeing themselves not as 'alcoholics' but as capable and worthwhile members of a society in which women are not only valued as sexual objects or as iconic homemakers but are seen as capable, hardworking, reliable and deserving of respect. WIAS aims to encourage women to continue discussion and socialising among themselves, as well as help with mentoring and networking, and introduce women to other local women's groups and organisations, according to their individual interests. To help in this, WIAS is developing a database of local organisations that are able to offer specialised help with self-harm, domestic abuse, homelessness etc, and will if required help women to access these on a one-to-one basis. The intention is that women will gain reliable support and access to different sources of support, all of which will both enrich their lives and make them more able to have confidence in their self-worth. In this way, WIAS will promote mutual respect and affirmation from others who have suffered the same condition – and recovered.

A social model of alcohol use

Another aspect of women's alcohol use that tends to be neglected in current services is the importance and relevance of context: that is, the factors that help women feel most safe and comfortable in discussing their issues – the time of day they can come; the choice to disclose or not to disclose personal details; the actual physical space; the sense of feeling welcomed and special. These are not easy to provide in mainstream treatment but could more easily take place in local community centres (ideally where there might also be other support services, including a crèche). There is much potential benefit in being able easily and safely to access non-judgemental support, without the need to go through a GP or make the journey to a specialised (and stigmatising) treatment centre. Such centres may not be the best place for some women.

> *High-cost intensive treatment programmes did not seem to produce better results than minimal interventions (Cameron, 1995: 45).*

> *Self-healing or spontaneous recovery from problem drinking is extremely common – up to three-quarters of those who have had a drinking problem take this route and, of these, up to two-thirds achieve moderation (Raistrick, Heather & Godfrey, 2006:173, referring to Klingemann, 2001).*

Furthermore, Galvani and Toft (2015) observe:

> *... some alcohol self-help groups can give messages about alcohol behaviour change that are unhelpful at best and dangerous at worst. Some treatment approaches based on 12 step or the Minnesota model, e.g. Alcoholics Anonymous, emphasise 'powerlessness' over alcohol as part of making changes to their drinking behaviour. They also suggest making amends to those who have been affected by the person's drinking. These types of concepts and suggested behaviour can be unhelpful to women who have suffered violence and abuse and who already feel powerless and have been blamed repeatedly for their partner's abuse of them.*

A very high proportion of women who identify with alcohol issues have experienced domestic abuse, often since childhood, although precise figures are difficult to obtain (Humphreys, Thiara & Regan, 2005; McKeganey et al, 2005).

It is crucial that all alcohol services recognise this and are trained to respond appropriately. It may not, for example, be in a woman's best interests to stop drinking before leaving a violent partner (Galvani & Humphreys, 2007).

> *Understanding women's drinking in context is not about offering causal explanations for the way women drink, but emphasises the diverse meanings and significance of this behaviour and how it interacts with other aspects of their lives (Barnes & Ward, 2015).*

Additionally, Hall (1994: 572) has noted that women may feel 'uncomfortable with AA's tendency to individualize problems, clothe recovery in the language of Christian spirituality, and encourage "surrender" and "powerlessness"'.

There are few mainstream services that offer such approaches, partly because of the medicalisation and diagnostic approach of mental health and addiction services, which categorise the individual by what is seen as the primary (medical) problem. In addition, other kinds of service provision, such as those dealing with homelessness, mental illness or sexual abuse, may be reluctant to try to help women who are still drinking. For example, some refuges providing shelter for women experiencing domestic abuse may be unable to accommodate a woman who is still drinking as they do not have the staff and other resources to provide sufficient support. While acknowledging the difficulties that many underfunded organisations may face, I suggest that they look seriously at the issues involved, and take steps towards providing more inclusive service provision wherever possible. This issue also has implications for commissioners and funders.

As I have suggested elsewhere:

> *The medical model of seeing alcohol 'abuse' as a disease of the will is widespread, while the failure of such an approach to produce change in individuals so afflicted is significant. The cost to society, in terms of physical health and emotional well-being, of incompetent 'treatment' and colossally expensive interventions, is enormous (Staddon, 2012: 201).*

A social model of alcohol use involves looking differently at the sources of distress; seeking them not in the individual psyche but in the very fabric of our society itself (Wilkinson & Pickett, 2009). In my own research women describe depression, sexual abuse, agonising childhood loss, loneliness and emotional deprivation as life experiences from which alcohol has provided some relief. It has been friend as well as foe, helping to cover over hidden grief and loss. WIAS aims to help women to overcome these disadvantages by understanding their causes and putting them in touch with appropriate help so that, ultimately, they no longer need this support. Small, friendly groups led by women who have survived 'alcoholism' are one route but other ideas are likely to come from the women themselves.

The politics of survivor-led solutions

As WIAS develops we shall be looking towards a future where, through networking with other third sector and public sector organisations, we shall be able to connect women with a variety of different forms of help for their needs, while listening to them and supporting them where they are at in the present. Our survivor perspective will help us to offer understanding and support, which are difficult to find elsewhere.

At the same time we will hope for political change whereby unequal social structures that contribute to mental distress and illness are identified and the worst inequalities addressed and, at the same time, the stigma for sufferers decreases. This, in turn, could lead both to savings in immediate costs and also longer-term benefits such as better health and welfare. There will, however, always be the danger that 'medical' approaches continue to be awarded greater significance and thus to carry more clout, even when they have been shown to be ineffectual or even damaging (Mann, 2012: 467).

Working to provide both a theoretical compass and a practical response is likely to mean a political battle with established views of alcohol use and with current theories of alcohol treatment, while demonstrating how these philosophies are grounded in established social expectations of a woman's role and perceptions of her self-worth.

Women's problematic alcohol use may be an expression of mental distress, but this distress is not 'only' personal; it is political (Radford, 1994). It is likely to be a consequence of being seen as a second sex (de Beauvoir, 1997) with fewer rights in many aspects of human life. It may be no accident that every woman I have interviewed in my research in connection with her alcohol use has named 'depression' as one of the root causes. I have drawn attention elsewhere (Staddon, 2013) to the way that alcohol services are permeated by a 'politics of recognition' (Lewis, 2009; Lewis, 2013):

> *... whereby respect and self-worth are withheld from those whose behaviour, whether caused by mental health issues, poverty, inequality or abuse, may cause the public to feel unsafe. Particularly of concern*

may be the behaviour of women, the mothers (and nurturers and life-long unpaid carers) of the next generation. If we drink, we are not acting as we are expected to behave; we have stepped outside 'normal behaviour' (Becker, 1966). We may be seen as a threat to the established order and perhaps to its view of morality (Staddon, 2014: 26).

It has meant that our small organisation has had to engage with issues of social justice. We are glad to help women to dress and heal their wounds but their pain and loss are the reasons we have felt impelled to publish, to seek audience with commissioners and health professionals, and to raise public awareness wherever possible of the inappropriateness, cruelty and inefficacy of current understandings of women's alcohol use.

A significant concern to the organisation's trustees is the difficulty we can envisage ahead as we acquire more funding and need to engage more with mainstream services and professions. Might we find ourselves drifting into professionalism and become merely an adjunct to the health services? Or will our board's feminist and service user ethos remain strong enough to counteract such a possibility?

References

Barnes M, Ward E (2015). Older women and alcohol. In: Staddon P (ed). *Women and Alcohol: social perspectives*. Bristol: Policy Press (pp103–118).

Barron JR (2004). *Struggle to Survive: challenges for delivering services on mental health, substance misuse and domestic violence*. Bristol: Women's Aid Federation of England.

Becker HS (1966). *Outsiders: studies in the sociology of deviance*. New York: The Free Press.

Cameron D (1995). *Liberating Solutions to Alcohol Concerns*. London: Jason Aronson Inc.

De Beauvoir S (1997, 1953 translation, 1945). *The Second Sex*. Reading: Vintage Classics.

Ettorre E (2007). *Revisioning Women and Drug Use: gender, power and the body*. Basingstoke: Palgrave MacMillan.

Fingarette H (1988). *Heavy Drinking: the myth of alcoholism as a disease*. Berkeley: University of California Press.

Galvani S, Humphreys C (2007). *The Impact of Violence and Abuse on Engagement and Retention Rates for Women in Substance Use Treatment: a report for the National Treatment Agency for Substance Misuse*. London: National Treatment Agency for Substance Misuse.

Galvani S with Toft C (2015). Domestic abuse and women's use of alcohol. In: Staddon P (ed). *Women and Alcohol: social perspectives*. Bristol: Policy Press (pp85-100).

Hall JM (1994). The experiences of lesbians in Alcoholics Anonymous. *Western Journal of Nursing Research 16*(5): 556–576.

Hall M, Bodenhamer B, Bolstad R, Hamblett M (2001). *The Structure of Personality: modelling 'personality' using*

NLP and neuro-semantics. Carmarthen: Crown House Publishing.

Humphreys C, Thiara RK, Regan L (2005). *Domestic Violence and Substance Use: overlapping issues in separate services? Final report to Home Office and the Greater London Authority*. London: the Stella Project.

International Centre for Drug Policy (2007). *Substance Misuse in the Undergraduate Medical Curriculum: a United Kingdom medical schools' collaborative programme*. London: The International Centre for Drug Policy (ICDP).

Lewis L (2009). Politics of recognition: what can a human rights perspective contribute to understanding users' experiences of involvement in mental health services? *Social Policy and Society 8*(2): 257–274.

Lewis L (2013). Recognition politics as a human rights perspective on service users' experiences of involvement in mental health services. In: Staddon P (ed). *Mental Health Service Users in Research: a critical sociological perspective*. Bristol: Policy Press (pp87–104).

Mann M (2012). *The Sources of Social Power. Vol. 2: the rise of classes and nation states, 1760-1914* (2nd edition). New York/Cambridge: Cambridge University Press.

McKeganey N, Neale J, Robertson M (2005). Physical and sexual abuse among drug users contacting drug treatment services in Scotland. *Drugs: Education, Prevention and Policy 12*(3): 223–232.

Moon L, Staddon P (2015). A drink in my hand: why 'putting down the glass' may be too simple a solution for lesbian women. In: Staddon P (ed). *Women and Alcohol: social perspectives*. Bristol: Policy Press (pp139–158).

Peele S (1995). *Diseasing of America: how we allowed recovery zealots and the treatment industry to convince us we are out of control*. Lexington, MA/San Francisco: Lexington Books/Jossey-Bass.

Radford J (1994). History of women's liberation movements in Britain: a reflective personal history. In: Griffin G, Hester M, Rai S, Roseneil S (ed). *Stirring It: challenges for feminism*. London: Taylor and Francis (pp40–58).

Raistrick D, Heather N, Godfrey C (2006). *Review of the Effectiveness of Treatment for Alcohol Problems*. London: National Treatment Agency for Substance Misuse.

Rogers C (1978). *On Personal Power: inner strength and its revolutionary impact*. London: Constable and Company Ltd.

Serrant L (2015). The silences in our dance: Black Caribbean Women and alcohol (mis)use. In: Staddon P (ed). *Women and Alcohol: social perspectives*. Bristol: Policy Press (pp119–138).

Shaw DL, McCombs M, Weaver DH, Hamm BJ (1999). Individuals, groups, and agenda melding: a theory of social dissonance. *International Journal of Public Opinion Research 11*(1): 2–24.

Staddon P (2005). Labeling out: the personal account of an ex-alcoholic lesbian feminist. *Journal of Lesbian Studies 9*(3): 69–78.

Staddon P (2009). *Making Whoopee? An exploration of understandings and responses around women's alcohol use*. PhD thesis. Plymouth: Plymouth University. Available at http://hdl.handle.net/10026.1/415 (accessed 12 November, 2015).

Staddon P (2012). No blame, no shame. Towards a social model of alcohol dependency: a story from emancipatory research. In: Carr S, Beresford P (eds). *Social Care, Service Users and User Involvement: building on research*. London: Jessica Kingsley Publishers (pp192–204).

Staddon P (2013). Theorising a social model of 'alcoholism': service users who misbehave. In: Staddon P (ed). *Mental Health Service Users in Research: a critical sociological perspective*. Bristol: Policy Press (pp105–120).

Staddon P (2014). Turning the tide. *Groupwork 24*(1): 26–41.

Tidmarsh J, Carpenter J, Slade J (2003). Practitioners as gatekeepers and researchers: family support outcomes. *International Journal of Sociology and Social Policy 23*(1-2): 59–79.

Vogt F, Hall S, Marteau T (2006). General practitioners' beliefs about effectiveness and intentions to recommend smoking cessation services: qualitative and quantitative studies. *BMC Family Practice 8*:39. http://www.biomedcentral.com/1471-2296/8/39 (accessed 12 November, 2015).

White WL (2008). *Recovery Management and Recovery-Oriented Systems of Care: scientific rationale and promising practices*. Pittsburgh, PA: Institute for Research, Education and Training in Addictions.

Wilkinson R, Pickett K (2010). *The Spirit Level: why equality is better for everyone*. London: Penguin Books.

14

Sexual violence in childhood: demarketing treatment options and strengthening our own agency

Zofia Rubinsztajn

This chapter has had a few false starts as I've found it hard to bring my thoughts together in a definite way. This is because for a number of years, often five days a week, I've been in the midst of what I'm trying to write about, and my views and feelings keep changing. I'm focusing on my work in one small organisation that started in Berlin 35 years ago. It was founded by ciswomen who had experienced sexual violence as children and openly identified as survivors of sexual abuse. To the present day, the project that I work on only employs survivors. We offer counselling to cisgender and transgender survivors, and to their significant others. We also offer support to professionals who encounter the topic of childhood sexual abuse in their work and seek our advice. A big part of our work involves giving support to the self-help groups that regularly meet on our premises. There are about 12 such groups held every week. Several years ago, the then workers changed the project's description from 'self-help' to a 'survivor-controlled' project.

But this chapter is not a statement on behalf of the project; what follows are solely my own reflections on four aspects of this unique response to sexual violence in childhood.

I

What I love and value about the framework of the project is that it explicitly welcomes and enables connections that go beyond the dominant understanding of how one should treat trauma survivors. When people come in for counselling, they're free to talk about whatever they find important; they're encouraged to find their own words, and nobody is going to stop them because of concerns about their mental health or the belief that they're not 'stable' enough to talk about traumatic experiences. Furthermore, nobody is going to ask them to seal away their painful memories in imaginary boxes that they can then kindly take back home with them. I think this is the most important thing: we're simply there to hear what the person has to say – we're invited to be their witness.

Many people come to us with the question of whether they even have the right to experience what happened to them as bad or hard to overcome. I value the fact that everybody has the chance to look for companionship in their personal journey. It's a journey that could potentially mean understanding themselves better, taking themselves seriously and reaching their own conclusions and decisions that will help them get where they want to be or make real what so far has been unimaginable. This might be about moving to another city, changing their name or legal status, including their sex, breaking contact with their family of origin, confronting an abuser and a great deal more.

What I often notice is how powerful it can be when people realise that *everybody* else in the project is a survivor. This happens particularly in the process of starting a self-help group. It's then, maybe for the first time, that the person is consciously in a space with other survivors and can physically grasp that they're not alone in their experience. This is very different from learning about the prevalence of sexual violence from statistics or reports that portray us as freaks in need of treatment. Instead you find yourself among likeable, tough and funny people who have gone through similar things and decided not to bear those experiences and their consequences on their own anymore, not to stay silent anymore. These are great moments that can change so much.

All this is the vital and precious side of the place where I work. So much is possible there, and it seems right to view this project as an alternative to mainstream services for trauma survivors. It is an alternative free of diagnoses with their narrow focus on individual pathologies, free of coercion and free of psychiatrists and therapists. As I have said, the concept for this alternative was grounded in the experiential knowledge and politicisation of a group of women who decided to openly identify as survivors of childhood sexual abuse. The women who founded the project were cisgendered and for the most part white Germans who shared the values and principles of Western feminism. More than 30 years later, aspects of the project's then self-image are no longer strived after, or at least they're not pursued by everybody. However, what certainly continues is the aspiration and commitment to doing things differently as survivors. But there is no such thing as a homogenous group of survivors. There is no big 'we'.

II

The founders of the organisation, like many other feminists, were certain about what the lives of women who had survived violence looked like and what exactly they needed. Furthermore, they shared firm stances on pornography, sex work and the use of alcohol and illegal drugs. The first two were simply to be abolished from society and the last two were – as is the norm elsewhere – grounds for exclusion as sobriety was a clear precondition for participating. The fact that women could be (and are) also abusers remained unspeakable for a long time. It disturbed the assumption that women-only spaces can be automatically assumed to be safe spaces. Broader social debates since then have resulted in significant changes to these views and also affected the project's approach. But these changes are often just talked about and have a role to play in the project's external image. They're not always truly taken forward and integrated in the day-to-day work.

So, for example, it's no longer the case that the salaried workers only come from the white German majority. And in the last couple of years transgender people have been able to access the project's structures and services. Given the organisation's history, this can be seen as a great step forward. But, if we consider the famous 'nothing about us without us' principle, then it makes no sense that transgender people are allowed to be service users and volunteers but explicitly denied the chance to become paid workers.

Further, it is no longer automatically assumed that women and transgender people who have experienced sexual violence only do sex work against their will or that women who wear a hijab do this only because they have to. But still the power of many unspoken norms and values can be keenly felt. It's no accident that sex workers only disclose their job in the context of individual counselling and don't feel confident to come out in group situations. Similarly, there are settings where people don't feel comfortable to share their experiences of racism and other discrimination. It also can't be said that these experiences never take place within the project itself. It's therefore not enough to declare 'transcultural competence' or a principle of non-discrimination in the statutes and other project materials.

Aside from all this, I would like to discuss one other issue that exemplifies the absence of a unifying 'we': I'm talking here about the different expectations and definitions of support of those who seek it out.

People who are familiar with the project's background and who explicitly opt for our services usually connect easily with what we're doing. They're not overstrained by the expectation that they should actively co-create the counselling framework, negotiate its terms and fill it with their own issues and needs. But these expectations are an obstacle for many others. This is especially true when people's life circumstances have not actually allowed their opinions to have any bearing. Ultimately this is the case for anyone who has been exposed to sexual violence, but survivors' biographies develop in a multitude of ways. Often people have grown used to the idea that, 'problematic' as they are, they will need several years of therapy and will never have a job, or at least not one they would want. They've been encouraged to accept that they will not lead a 'normal' life. The more this is internalised, the more surprised people are when they find themselves in a counselling situation where none of this is assumed. People who learned that they self-harm because they suffer from a personality disorder are invited to think about the personal meaning that self-harm has for them. This shift can overwhelm people to the point that they never come back, or return only after a couple of years.

It should be said that it's not only in psychiatry that people's experiences are pathologised and overwritten. Anti-violence projects such as women's shelters, counselling centres and hotlines are now also increasingly establishing separate services for the 'mentally ill'. With the help of specialised training, or by collecting and collating the available psychiatric 'expert' materials (such as psychoeducation), these projects are trying to gain greater professional competence in dealing with 'difficult' women. As a result, they lose sight of the fact that these women's reactions and ways of being in the world make sense, are understandable in light of the violence they experienced, and are in no way symptoms of a 'disorder'. What is needed here is not more funding and staff, as is often argued, but a willingness to provide actual support rather than changing the focus and producing more special needs.

However, the fact is that some abuse survivors do conceive of themselves primarily as individuals in need of treatment. They see our project as another place where they can go, in addition to therapeutic and psychiatric services, in part to unload everything they dislike about those services. Some people simply believe in the need to structure the day, making appointments everywhere just to get through the time and treating us as their waste bin. Personally, I am not a good counterpart for people who explicitly demand that somebody else manages their life. The thought of meeting these expectations disturbs me; in fact it strikes me as quite obscene.

Thinking more broadly, I would argue that, if projects like the one I am describing start adjusting their overall approach in order to uncritically serve all expectations, then our work will become somewhat vague and random. Furthermore, this vagueness will be a disservice to the people who want to make use of our project as it was conceived. After all, the project exists for people who are looking for a particular kind of framework and who are not well served by social work or therapeutic or psychiatric services. Our project is one of the rare spaces for people who want to deal with their own histories in a self-determined way and at their own pace, deciding for themselves how much they want to disclose. Our concept of support speaks to people who want to be challenged and bring their own agenda to counselling, self-help groups or other forums. Broadening our 'target' group to include those who claim special rights and primarily understand themselves as traumatised victims would mean we would lose the space that was hard to establish – a space for survivors who want to co-create and take full responsibility for their own actions.

III

Thinking about the future of survivor-founded, grassroots spaces, I believe that it is not enough to base these spaces on the idea of a shared identity. What emerges is always about different people in different realities, with different values and views. It is crucial to acknowledge and allow those differences. It is crucial to let them speak and let them be.

However, I also ask myself why, in survivor projects such as this, a smaller group often emerges and that group suddenly begins to dominate and talk in the name of everybody else. Why is it that one exclusive circle of people discusses and defines the right and wrong that should then become valid for everybody? I think about this a lot and notice that these dominant groups often contain people who profit from keeping things as they are, who enjoy their privileges and have strong needs to assert themselves and get the same importance and recognition as professionals. These people seek acknowledgment and appreciation from those they claim to criticise and from whom they say they want to distance themselves. This kind of professional recognition can become one of the project's goals, often hidden behind a firm set of rules or behind prescriptions about what is and isn't feasible in its day-to-day work.

This is when the space that was once meant to be alternative starts to resemble what we know of conventional services. If a person in a mad state of mind has an appointment at 2.00pm but arrives instead at 4.00pm, we can, of course, say they are too late and send them away. We can claim this is legitimate. But this then completely misses the point that I personally find essential in these situations: because of their lateness, this person will not make it anywhere on time all day; they will be two hours late everywhere. This suggests that they will not be able to talk to anybody for the entire day. This is why making space for flexibility is important. But not all my colleagues are willing to provide these kinds of apparently unreasonable adjustments. Willingness to improvise and rearrange because this is needed at a particular moment can lead to accusations of acting unprofessionally and against the rules. Even if the notion of '(un-) professionalism' is not spelled out, you can feel that it is being implied. In fact, what is required is the recognition that this is a way of handling a concrete situation and not an issue for theoretical debate.

Such strictness and belief in the value of a preset structure recall the rules of psychiatric services, but those who insist on this approach do not notice this. I know that in our project we are capable of flexibility and have rarely experienced situations where things are non-negotiable. Even a person who arrives two hours late understands that they are off-schedule; I can tell them that I am not able to sit with them for too long and have other things to do but that they can have a coffee in the kitchen or smoke a cigarette now that they have finally arrived.

There are many things that are not provided for because they don't seem to fit within the work framework. What I'm concerned about are all the situations where something other than counselling is needed. There are, for instance, situations where a person says that they need to completely disconnect from their current life in order to have a life at all. Such a person may have a sudden need for support with things they cannot do on their own, such as moving house. If we take seriously the fact that they don't want to ask for support from those who damaged them then practical aid has to be provided. Even if this is not typical in a counselling framework, I think taking care of such things is part of a project of this kind. This does not mean taking everything over; it can mean, for example, making an effort to find volunteers to help with the move. I personally find deeply problematic arguments that this kind of practical support cannot be part of our work because it is trivial or apparently goes too far.

IV

Having now been intensively involved in several projects, I am not certain how we can prevent 'survivor-control' from being turned into a label that can sell anything, including the kind of mainstream help I wouldn't wish on anybody.

When we find ourselves in a psychiatric or similarly oppressive system, we know where we are and can position ourselves. An alternative framework that holds the promise of something completely different but doesn't feel the way it should can make us doubt our own senses and perceptions. This is particularly bad when these alternative frameworks target people whose nightmares are rooted in precisely this phenomenon.

My wish is that those of us who don't want to settle for fake alternatives, who are not intent on establishing something at any cost, can draw on our peculiarity and never accept that anything is impossible. My wish is that we can empower each other to keep on searching for more.

15

The personal ombudsman: an example of supported decision-making

Maths Jesperson

Our personal ombudsman service in Skåne (PO-Skåne) has become well known all over the world as one of the few concrete examples of what is now called 'supported decision-making' that meets the requirements of the UN Convention on the Rights of Persons with Disabilities (CRPD) (United Nations, 2006).

Article 12 of the Convention clearly states that all forms of guardianship contravene the rights of disabled people and should be abolished. Societies should provide the necessary support so that people who have difficulties expressing themselves or communicating are able to make their own decisions. Their right to make decisions about their lives should not be taken away and handed over to another person (such as a guardian or a psychiatrist) but should always remain with the person themselves, although some may need some support to express and communicate their decisions. 'Substituted decision-making' should be abolished and replaced by 'supported decision-making'.

Our experience at PO-Skåne proves that it is possible to fulfil this requirement of the CRPD, and that it is not just a utopian idea.

Because it is so unique, there is great interest in this model, with many countries considering abolishing their old guardianship systems. But our service started 10 years before the UN Convention was adopted, and in another context: it emerged from the experience of users and survivors of psychiatry, and our ideas about the support we felt we might need in certain situations.

The origins of PO-Skåne

The Swedish service user organisation RSMH (the Swedish National Association for Social and Mental Health) was founded in 1967, when the old asylum system in Sweden was at its peak, with a total of 36,000 inmates in its long-stay psychiatric hospitals. This peak was also a turning point, because soon afterwards the process of closing down the big mental hospitals began, and RSMH was one of the driving forces behind this reform. When psychiatric patients started to live in the community instead of in hospitals, RSMH acquired a new role, alongside its more political one – namely, peer support.

By the end of the 1980s RSMH had grown into a vast organisation, with 8,000 members in 150 local groups and 100 former psychiatric patients employed full-time, with their salaries subsidised by the government. Many of the groups had big premises and even houses of their own that served as drop-in and activity centres and were run by the psychiatric users themselves. We started self-help groups and dialogue forums, but above all we supported our members in all kinds of situations – from dealing with very practical matters to managing episodes of distress, suicidality and madness.

Although we had considerable resources, they were not enough. There were constraints to the peer support we could offer in terms of how many people we could help, the legal expertise we could provide, the amount of time we could offer and so on. Furthermore, it was easy to provide peer support for psychiatric patients who were your friends and whom you liked. But what were we to do with those we didn't like or those we experienced as annoying or aggressive? Who was supposed to support them?

In 1995 an opportunity emerged to apply for government funding for pilot personal ombudsman (PO) projects. We saw this as an opportunity to take our experience of peer support a step further. The Swedish system of POs emerged from the psychiatric reform of 1995. The parliamentary committee preparing the reform had noticed that something essential was missing in the support of people with psychiatric problems in the community, but they had only a very vague notion of what that should be. They thought that there should be someone to help people with severe psychosocial disabilities achieve what they needed and wanted, and came up with the totally new idea of a 'personal ombudsman' (in Swedish, *personligt ombud*). But they didn't come up with much more than that.

In order to develop this new idea, the Swedish parliament decided to fund 10 different PO projects over three years, 1995–1998. They discussed at length who should run the new services. Some thought that it should be the government, others that such services should be run by independent organisations, to avoid conflicts of interest. The role of PO was compared with that of lawyers, who must be independent if they are to be able to defend their clients. Because of these conflicting opinions, the parliament decided to trial different models for the PO services, with different governance arrangements, over the three years.

This seemed to me to be a good opportunity for RSMH to develop a PO model of our own. I wrote an application for funding, and our project was one of the 10 selected, although the National Health Board received hundreds of applications. Our project was one of only two that were led by a service user organisation. All the other pilot projects were run by local authorities.

The PO system is not the same as peer support, but it is based on many of the fundamental principles of peer support. The idea fitted very well with my own experience and thinking, and especially my own model, the Jungle Model (Jesperson, 1995).

The Jungle Model

This model emerged from my own hard experience of coming out of madness – which didn't mean getting back to 'normal life', but moving forward to a new life. During my own journey I got much inspiration and insight from authors like Jung and Laing, from the big, universal stories in the Bible, like the crossing of the Red Sea in the Old Testament, and especially from the writings of the great Catholic mystic Juan de la Cruz (1542–1591).

In all this I was supported by a retired psychiatrist, Stephan Mark-Vendel, who was completely on my side and who confirmed that I was on the right path. He was an unusual psychiatrist who, after his retirement, denounced the medical model that he had been following his whole career and, in older age, returned to university to study hypnosis. He was in many ways an old-fashioned doctor, but at the same time very open to the whole spectrum of expressions of human spirituality: for example, he experienced premonitions himself. Most importantly, he fully supported me, never denying my experiences or my own interpretations of them, never calling them a mental illness, but regarding them as real, and trying to help me find out their meaning and the direction I had to take.

Stephan is for me the prototype for the kind of support you need when you are in a difficult phase of your life. I learned a lot from him and have used that learning during my 30 years of peer support in the user movement.

In the Jungle Model I use the jungle as a metaphor for madness. The jungle is a dangerous place, with no paths to follow and no maps to guide you; a place where you are surrounded by wild animals and many traps. Once you have entered it, it's hard to find the way out, and there is always a risk you will be lost in it for ever. There is no way back so you must try to find your way out the other side. It's good to have a companion on this journey. I don't mean an expert who knows the way out, but four eyes see more than two, and it's good to have someone to discuss your thoughts and ideas with while walking. This companion shouldn't try to pull you out of the jungle, which is impossible. Instead he should enter the jungle himself and make his way to the place where you are, even if this is a reality unknown to him. The main task for the companion is to accept your experience, to dialogue with it – and to start the journey out of the jungle from there.

I have never transferred the Jungle Model to the PO system, which is more concrete and practical. But the way the POs have to work puts them in the same position as the companions in my Jungle Model, and in their work you see them following the same approach.

Establishing PO-Skåne

RSMH launched the project in its regional branch in Skåne, with two full-time POs and me, as the project manager, in 1995. Both ombudsmen were members of our organisation and had experience of depression and psychosis and of being psychiatric patients, but above all they had professional skills in dealing with authorities and legal matters. One of them was a trained social worker and the other had completed a degree in theology. They could give both personal and professional support. The project drew on our experience and knowledge of peer support to establish the fundamental principles for how the two POs should work.

In 2000 we transformed the pilot project into the permanent service, run by a new non-governmental organisation, PO-Skåne. Skåne is the most southern province of Sweden, with about 1.2 million inhabitants. One third live in Malmö, which is the third largest city in Sweden. PO-Skåne now has contracts with 15 local governments in Skåne – both in cities as well as in very rural areas.

PO-Skåne is run by RSMH and the family support organisation IFS (the Schizophrenia Fellowship). Half of the board is appointed by RSMH and the other half by IFS, which means that the board largely consists of users and family members. The board is the employer of the managing director and the 18 POs. This means that, although PO-Skåne is a professional service, it is user controlled and user run. The board members are volunteers but the director and the POs are salaried. The service is free for clients.

How PO-Skåne operates

It's hard to translate the Swedish word *'personligt ombud'* into English. The most accurate translation is probably 'personal agent', but I usually translate it as 'personal ombudsman' so I can use the same abbreviation, PO, in English as in Swedish. The term 'personal ombudsman' has now become the established translation, and has been used in numerous international publications.

Most of the POs are trained social workers, but some also have a background in law. It is important for the POs to have a very good knowledge of law and the legal system, as well as public administration and the way the authorities work. Because this knowledge is so crucial, we prefer to employ people who have academic qualifications in these fields. The other attributes we are looking for are their attitude towards clients and their ability to communicate. These are personal qualities and cannot really be learned through any training. To ensure that the new POs have the qualities we want, they serve a six-month probationary period.

It is not difficult to recruit new POs. Most of our applicants are women in their 40s. They often say that this is the way of working that they have dreamt of all their lives; that this was why they wanted to become social workers in the first place, but instead found themselves caught in a bureaucratic system, focusing solely on decisions about money.

The personal satisfaction for the PO themselves in this new job is that they develop close relationships with their clients and are able to work with them over a long period. This makes it possible for them to see that what they do does make a difference: that it transforms people's lives in a positive direction. One of our POs, Henrik Lundius, puts it this way: 'You meet fantastic people all the time. It's fun to fight for something good. This is the only job where you leave your home in the morning and you actually do good.'

For their first few months the new PO is assigned an experienced mentor. He or she also attends a programme of workshops, seminars and lectures to train them in their new role. One of the most important things is to unlearn their old profession as a social worker or lawyer. They are not supposed to bring their previous roles into this new role. A new PO starts with only one or two clients and isn't expected to take on a full caseload (approximately 15 to 20 clients) until several months later.

A PO works only on the instructions of their client; they do only what their client wants them to do. They are not in any kind of alliance with psychiatry or social services or any other authority, or with the client's relatives or other contacts. It can take a long time – sometimes several months – before clients know and feel able to say what kind of help they want, so the PO has to wait, even if a lot of things in the client's life are chaotic and in a mess. This means that the PO has to develop a long-term relationship with their clients, usually over several years. This is a necessary condition if a trusting relationship is to be developed that enables the client then to address more essential matters.

In our service the most important goal has been to develop ways of working that are acceptable to people with the most difficult mental health problems. In other projects it is usually the clients who have to adjust to the bureaucratic system, but we work in the opposite way: the POs have to be very flexible, creative and unconventional in finding ways to work with their clients.

Some working principles

We consider the following principles to be necessary in order to truly reach the clients and practise supported decision-making with them.

- The PO doesn't work weekday office hours only. There are seven days in the week and 24 hours in each day. The PO must be ready to work at all hours because their clients' problems don't only happen within office hours and some clients are easier to contact at evenings and weekends. The PO is contracted to work 40 hours a week but creates a flexible working schedule each week, built around their clients' needs.

- The PO isn't office based, because offices equate with power. The PO works from their own home, with the help of a telephone and the internet. They meet their clients at the client's home or at neutral places in town.

- The PO works primarily to a relationship model. As many clients are very suspicious or hostile towards the authorities, or hard to reach for other reasons, the PO has to go out and find them. Reaching clients involves several steps: making contact; developing communication; establishing a relationship; starting a dialogue, and getting commissions from the client. Each of these steps can take a long time to achieve. Just making contact can sometimes take several months. It can mean going out and talking to a homeless person in a park, or speaking through the letter box to someone who won't let anyone into their home. But it's only when the relationship is established and a dialogue has begun that the PO can receive commissions from their client.

- People should not have to go through any bureaucratic process to get a PO. Many psychiatric patients would be put off if they had to sign any forms or get a formal referral, and they would probably be the people who need a PO most. There's no formal procedure for getting a PO from PO-Skåne. Once a relationship is established the PO just asks, 'Do you want me to be your PO?' If the answer is 'yes', the whole thing is settled. And it can be terminated just as easily.

- The PO should be able to support the client with any kind of issue. The client's priorities are unlikely to be the same as the priorities of the authorities or relatives. Our experience suggests that the client's first priorities are not usually housing or work but existential questions such as, 'What's the point of my life? Why has my life become the life of a mental patient? What hope do I have for change?', and issues around sexuality and problems with family relationships. A PO must be prepared to spend a lot of time talking with their client about these kinds of issues – not just fix practical problems.

- A PO should be very skilled in advocating for the client's rights with the authorities and in court.

- The client has the right to stay anonymous. If they don't want anyone to know they have a PO, this must be respected. PO-Skåne receives funding from the municipality for the service but there is a paragraph in the contract that says that the PO does not have to disclose the name of the client.

- The PO doesn't keep any records. All papers relating to their work together belong to the client. When their relationship with a client ends, the PO has either to return all papers to the client or burn them, in the presence of the client. They should keep no papers or notes.

Fifteen years on

Now, 15 years later, we have 310 POs in Sweden providing supported decision-making for more than 6,000 individuals. A total of 245 municipalities – 84 per cent of all the municipalities in Sweden – include POs in their social services. In 2013 new directives came into force that enshrine the PO system in the national welfare structure.

The PO system is also saving considerable amounts of money for the government. Studies show that PO work reduces costs by approximately €80,000 per assisted person over a five-year period. For every euro spent on the PO system, the government gets €17 back. So it also makes good economic sense.

The municipalities can choose to run the PO service themselves or they can contract a voluntary sector organisation to run it for them. We think it's important that the PO service is independent from the government in order to avoid conflicts of interest and to gain the trust of the people who need the service most.

Internationally there is great interest in PO-Skåne and the Swedish PO system, mainly in connection with the CRPD. When countries are implementing the CRPD they have to meet the requirements of Article 12 to replace 'substituted decision-making' (guardianship) with 'supported decision-making'. But worldwide there are few examples of how this actually works.

There is also great interest outside of the context of the CRPD. We are often met with an enthusiastic response when we present PO-Skåne at international meetings. One elderly facilitator at a conference in Lisbon became so enthusiastic on hearing about PO-Skåne that he stepped forward and exclaimed to the audience: 'This is revolutionary! This is earthshaking!'

References

Jesperson M (1995). Die befreiung von der psychiatrischen diagnostik durch selbsthilfe. In: Bock T, Buck D, Gross J (eds). *Abschied von Babylon: verständigung über grenzen in der psychiatrie*. Bonn: Psychiatrie Verlag (pp195–200).

United Nations (2006). *Convention on the Rights of Persons with Disabilities*. New York: United Nations.

16

Kindred Minds: a personal perspective

Renuka Bhakta

Our visions of a better future are often born from a sense of social injustice, the need for change and an unswerving belief that a different kind of world is possible. My father tells how, when he was 10, he was lifted onto the shoulders of his father to see Mohandas Gandhi leading huge crowds in peaceful protest against the infamous Salt Tax imposed by the British in colonial India (Kuhn, 2010). As my father stood with his father, singing protest songs in unison with the crowd, he glimpsed *satyagraha* in action. That is, people standing peacefully together to highlight injustice and try to create a fairer world. I believe that such memories, my dad's strong principles and the way he has lived his life instilled in me, from an early age, a deep awareness of political and social injustice, the power of proactive collective action and (within that) the importance of individual relationships. All of this has influenced the way I think and act, and never more so than when I became involved in Kindred Minds, a project specifically designed to address the concerns of mental health system survivors from Black and minority ethnic (BME) communities in and around the London Borough of Southwark, one of the most ethnically diverse areas in London.[1]

---

1. In this chapter, familiar (but often contested) terminology has been used in the following way:
   - survivor – someone who has experience of being in the mental health system and surviving
   - BME – people from Black and minority ethnic communities/backgrounds
   - Black – a political term to denote those who are discriminated against on the basis of their skin colour, who feel solidarity with one another because of this experience but who may have very different cultural backgrounds.

Having got caught up in the mental health system myself, I had seen firsthand the oppressive ways in which that system can crush people, particularly those from Black communities. I had always known about the effects of personal and institutionalised racism in society generally, but seeing this reproduced so harshly in the mental health services had a profound effect on me. When the chance arose for me to become involved in Kindred Minds, I jumped at it, seeing it as an opportunity to raise the concerns of Black survivors, consider them in broad sociopolitical as well as mental health contexts and demand service improvements through proactive collective action.

The birth of Kindred Minds

Kindred Minds was born in 2007, in relatively positive national and local contexts. Nationally, the UK government was finally acknowledging the existence of race inequalities in mental health and the need to seriously address them. Issues about racism and stereotyping in psychiatry had been raised as early as the1980s (Fernando, 2012) but it was not until 2005 that the government made a commitment to specifically focus on this. Sparked by the public inquiry into the death of David 'Rocky' Bennett (a young Black man who died while being restrained on a psychiatric ward) and its explicit criticism of mental health services (Norfolk, Suffolk and Cambridgeshire Strategic Health Authority, 2003), the government introduced a national five-year programme entitled 'Delivering Race Equality' (Department of Health, 2005). For many Black survivors and their communities, this programme seemed like a real breakthrough, offering hope to those whose lives had been damaged by the mental health services purporting to care for them.

At a local level, mental health services and voluntary organisations were (in line with government policy) also focusing on race and mental health in a range of ways. The local Mind organisation in Southwark (one of the few survivor-led ones in the country) had been concerned for some time about issues of race and racism in mental health services. They were seeing how Black people were very over-represented in local mental health services yet under-represented in community organisations such as their own. Mindful of their responsibility to local BME survivors, the leadership in Southwark Mind knew they had to reach out to this constituency and applied for funding to develop a specific BME project. Probably because of its well-established reputation as a genuinely survivor-led organisation, its strong record of campaigning and solid infrastructure, Southwark Mind was awarded funding for three years and the scene was set for Kindred Minds to be born.

I was one of the few BME members of Southwark Mind at the time and had previously worked with them as a volunteer on several generic projects. When I was approached to help in setting up a new project, I was at a point in my life where, in order to stay out of the system, I needed to begin to acknowledge and address my own issues of race and identity. I was also aware that focusing specifically on BME issues would involve working in a way that I hadn't previously done with Southwark Mind, which was a predominately White organisation. It would mean highlighting the differences in my own cultural upbringing and require me to nurture a stronger sense of my identity and carve a space as an Indian woman, born and raised in the UK. I had already explored some of this at a more personal level, most recently through my involvement in re-evaluation counselling. This was giving me an understanding of how change at a personal level can be neither meaningful nor lasting without involving change on a societal level (Jackins, 1994). It was clear to me that becoming involved in the Kindred Minds project would allow me to explore whether I could, within the Southwark Mind user-led model, meaningfully set up and sustain a BME project whose aim was not only to empower individual lives but to set a precedent for improving mental health services on a wider level. I knew I had the values, knowledge, skills, personal qualities and courage needed to be usefully involved and had also developed strong support around me, particularly from key individuals in Southwark Mind and my re-evaluation counselling communities and within my spiritual context. All of this, coupled with my fierce determination not to be drawn back to the mental health system, felt very positive and I stepped into Kindred Minds with optimism and hope, albeit also with a little apprehension.

The development of Kindred Minds

When I first got involved, in 2006, I worked as a volunteer, helping with the conceptualisation of this yet unnamed BME project. In 2007 I was recruited as one of three development workers. Having spent 10 years ineffectively grappling with the mental health system, this was a pivotal turning point for me. I had been unemployed, lacking in confidence, within a psychiatric system that told me something was wrong with me, and frightened of moving away from the tenuous security of the benefits system, not knowing whether I might end up in 'relapse'. Working at Kindred Minds meant that I took on a paid work routine, enabling me to manage my household and financial duties. It also meant that I held a position with responsibility and professional status with outside agencies, and was able to work with people with similar experiences to me. Although these changes were a big leap into the unknown, it was probably the most supportive environment in which I could take this plunge. With my two inspiring and committed colleagues, we launched and began to develop what became Kindred Minds, guided by the previously untapped resourcefulness and collective wisdom of BME survivors who approached us and then became active members. This gradually created a vibrant and exciting group whose progress and achievements can perhaps best be summarised as follows:

- we got Kindred Minds known both locally and nationally as a credible, survivor-led project
- we built trust and positive relationships with local BME survivors and learned firsthand what their concerns about mental health were and what they saw as solutions, and developed our activities accordingly
- we enabled BME survivors to raise awareness of their concerns and work collectively to get them addressed.

One of our proudest achievements was the role we played in saving a South Asian mental health drop-in service (Amardeep) from threatened closure by the local mental health trust. We helped by organising capacity-building events and meetings, public demonstrations with media coverage and formal meetings with decision makers from the local trust and by encouraging Amardeep members to keep the campaign going. By overcoming many hurdles, Amardeep was eventually able to stop the proposed closure of their service and it is still active seven years on.

We also achieved other successes, not necessarily laid out in our funding bid but absolutely crucial to the way we worked and to our philosophy in Kindred Minds. We maintained our BME autonomy under the umbrella of a predominantly White organisation, developed ourselves as a completely genuine BME survivor-led project, established an effective Kindred Minds staff team and evolved into a creative BME project that could explore and offer some alternatives and a non-medical approach to mental health. Interestingly, these were the areas where we faced our greatest challenges but we were able to acknowledge and address them and use them as valuable learning opportunities.

The challenges

Inevitably, we faced a number of challenges as we sought to develop Kindred Minds according to our principles and vision.

Maintaining Kindred Minds' autonomy

Kindred Minds' genesis within Southwark Mind and their role as our umbrella organisation inevitably caused cynicism among some BME survivors who thought that Southwark Mind was simply 'jumping onto the national Delivering Race Equality bandwagon'. I felt some sympathy with this view but, having previously worked successfully with Southwark Mind, I felt that developing Kindred Minds with them was a risk worth taking. It felt that the task of our team was to acknowledge the concerns of BME users while at the same time showing faith in Southwark Mind and its stated commitment to letting Kindred Minds develop in its own way, without trying to control it. We tried to do this by giving examples of Southwark Mind's survivor-empowering work and their good practice with marginalised/seldom-heard groups. But we were well aware that trust takes time to build, so we tried not to be too pushy and to take gentle steps instead. We needed to let members experience for themselves how the partnership was working and then make up their own minds.

The question was also raised as to why we needed to come under an umbrella organisation at all and why we could not simply be independent. We knew from other projects how difficult it would be for Kindred Minds to establish and sustain itself from scratch so we agreed with members to set independence as a long-term goal, and in the meantime to build firm foundations on which to grow. Interestingly, once Kindred Minds became established, Southwark Mind's umbrella involvement was rarely raised as an issue. However we, the staff of Kindred Minds, knew how much the leadership in Southwark Mind were doing behind the scenes to enable us to focus on our crucial work with Kindred Minds members.

Concerns about the relationship between Kindred Minds and Southwark Mind were not confined to Kindred Minds and its members. Some members of Southwark Mind expressed anxieties and it felt crucial to bring them on board. We therefore organised a BME survivor-led workshop as a safe environment where we could engage in open dialogue about race and particular issues for BME survivors. This was a huge step that I had personally wanted to take for a long time and, empowered by the opportunity, I was able to raise issues that I had never heard openly discussed before. To Southwark Mind's credit, its members generally seemed willing to explore and debate the issues, with discussions continuing outside the workshop and both sides trying to keep open the channels of communication and make race an acceptable and informative topic to talk about. Nurturing such mutually respectful openness helped dispel many fears and suspicions, and I feel it helped create an environment where Kindred Minds and Southwark Mind could work constructively together, with each retaining its values and autonomy in its own way.

A genuine BME survivor-led and run project

Many projects claim the title of 'user/survivor led' but, while they may consult with users/survivors, we are rarely involved in genuine decision-making. We knew right from the start that we wanted to be different, to go beyond consultation and involve members in more meaningful ways. To us, being survivor-led meant explicitly valuing the knowledge, skills, interests and creativity that survivors brought, and using these to organically shape the project. We knew we had to prioritise BME survivors' issues and concerns and be accountable to them in very transparent ways while at the same time satisfying the requirements of our funders. Bringing survivors together and nurturing relationships and group cohesion were essential to this work. Personally, I needed to use a way of working that felt natural to me and would enable me to go at an appropriate pace and was not too pushy. I used key co-counselling techniques (listening and giving attention) as a basis, which enabled mutually supportive and sustainable relationships to develop in authentic ways. We in the staff team had to rapidly learn when and how to stand back and enable others to come forward, but also recognise when it was important to take a lead. We had to develop a co-operative way of working that responded to members and allowed a sharing of power and authority. Examples of this coming to fruition were when Kindred Minds members played a major role in organising and running two successful pan-London, BME survivor-only conferences, the first called 'Doing it for Ourselves' and the second 'Get To Know Us First'.

Of course, it was not always sweetness and light. How could it be when survivors coming to Kindred Minds had experienced harsh treatment and racism not only from the mental health system but from society too? Sometimes there were eruptions because of heightened emotions and, while this was always acknowledged, there was also a need to set boundaries, resolve conflicts quickly and effectively and maintain order. Although we did this in a fairly formal way, members seemed to appreciate the way we set things out clearly and helped create a sense of safety.

Establishing a strong worker team

In order for Kindred Minds to function effectively, the three development workers had to work together as a cohesive team. This could have been challenging, given that we were each different in terms of our life and mental health experiences and our views on how services needed to be changed. We had to learn to work positively with this diversity, which proved invaluable when it came to working with people of many different backgrounds who would became involved with Kindred Minds. The three of us also brought a diversity of knowledge, skills and abilities to the team and we used these to develop a way of working that not only played to our individual strengths but also enabled us to learn from one another in constructive and non-competitive ways. Each of us was trying to get into the routine of work after varying periods of time in the mental health system. Southwark Mind's understanding and experience of working with such personal circumstances proved invaluable. I feel that working through these challenges enabled us to establish a successful, non-hierarchical, cohesive and mutually enabling team that was able to work effectively with each other and the diversity of Kindred Minds members.

Alternative and non-medical approaches

One of Kindred Minds' key aims was to provide opportunities for BME survivors to take responsibility for their wellbeing through creative thinking and by offering non-medical alternatives that they might want to consider. We provided complementary therapies at all our activities (including campaigning) and this became our trademark, allowing survivors to discover what was useful for them personally. For many, Kindred Minds was the first group they had been involved in outside of the mental health system, and sometimes it took time to adapt to our non-medical culture. The challenge here was that some of us had very strong views, particularly around psychotropic drugs, but found that these were not always shared by our members. We had to learn to accept this and respect survivors' rights to their own views, to hold back on the passion we felt and make a conscious decision as to whether to provide information, challenge or keep silent about contentious issues.

In line with our non-medical approach, we tried to do away with the trappings of the mental health system, which so often puts people in boxes and restricts their potential. We were open access – no referrals, no budget payments, no case workers or case notes. We wanted anyone who self-identified as a BME survivor/user to become involved in Kindred Minds in ways that felt comfortable for them. People came for a whole range of reasons, from simply wanting a place to be and some social interaction to wanting to take on the world and fight against social injustice and race inequalities. All played a part in creating and shaping Kindred Minds into what I believe was a very unique and successful project.

Lessons learned

I left Kindred Minds in February 2014, although I am still in touch with the users who came together through the project and who continue to meet, with very little funding. I gained much valuable learning through my involvement in the development of Kindred Minds. First, the experience of being a (involuntary) mental health patient and losing my sense of control brought unexpected learning. I found that other survivors had similar experiences and decided to learn more about this, and I used the information to regain my sense of power and autonomy and used this in my work to improve current mental health services.

I also learnt the value and importance of building and relying on a wider network and resources, as well as the vital importance of trusting my own judgements and developing my ability to think and take action. That process of making mistakes, failing, working out what went wrong and trying again was essential if I was to have even a remote chance of success.

Finally, through all of this I have understood at a much deeper level how society is organised, both historically and financially, where oppressed people uphold a capitalist system that supports the few rich. I have also learned what it means to build trust and find allies we can really rely on.

Postscript

> *It's the action, not the fruit of the action, that's important. It may not be in your power, may not be in your time, that there'll be any fruit. But that doesn't mean you stop doing the right thing. You may never know what results come from your action. But if you do nothing, there will be no result. (Mohandas Gandhi)*

By the end of 2010, the national sociopolitico environment around race and mental health had changed. Delivering Race Equality had ended unsatisfactorily, with many people (including those in Kindred Minds) disillusioned that it had not fulfilled its potential (RAWOrg, 2011). Furthermore, the initiative that had been sparked by the death of a young Black man while he was being restrained on a psychiatric ward ended, ominously, with the death of yet another young Black man, Olaseni Lewis, in similar circumstances. 2010 also saw the introduction of a single Equality Act that replaced all the previous separate equalities legislation and took the focus off race. In addition, the global recession had kicked in and drastic cuts in funding meant race no longer seemed to be a priority. All this inevitably impacted on the morale of BME survivors, and Kindred Minds members struggled to keep their hopes alive. Southwark Mind, because of its own internal challenges, was no longer able to provide Kindred Minds with managerial support. However, in spite of these difficulties, we managed to acquire funding to continue. The challenges now were very different, largely because of changes in national and local contexts and priorities. But Kindred Minds, with support from its members, continued to develop and in many ways flourish. Kindred Minds has now moved into its third phase of development, the passion, resilience, commitment and strength of its members collectively carrying it onwards and upwards.

Being involved in Kindred Minds was exciting, inspirational and revealing on both personal and professional levels. Usually when I write about Kindred Minds, it's been about statistics, achieving pre-set outcomes, accountability to the funders and value for money. Here I've had the opportunity to be more real, presenting Kindred Minds' many strengths, huge potential and positive achievements, but also the challenges and external pressures, which were at times very demanding. I guess this reflects how life has been for many of us BME survivors – a journey of promise and possibility too often interrupted by forces beyond our control. Yet, somehow the spirit survives, as when people who have been through such experiences come together in more enabling and empowering circumstances. Kindred Minds was by no means perfect, but for many of us it was crucially important. I continue to personally benefit from the many lessons I learned at Kindred Minds. Maybe we haven't changed the world, but at least we stand up with pride and take action.

Acknowledgements

I wish to thank Premila Trivedi and Yan Weaver, who have helped me write this chapter and supported me throughout my time with Kindred Minds.

References

Department of Health (2005). *Delivering Race Equality in Mental Health Care: an action plan for reform inside and outside services and the Government's response to the independent inquiry into the death of David Bennett*. London: Department of Health.

Jackins H (1994). *How 'Re-evaluation Counseling' Began*. Seattle: Rational Island Publishers.

Kuhn B (2010). *The Force Born of Truth: Mohandas Gandhi and the Salt March*. Minneapolis, MN: Twenty-First Century Books.

Norfolk, Suffolk and Cambridgeshire Strategic Health Authority (2003). *Independent Inquiry into the Death of David Rocky Bennett*. Chair: Sir John Blofeld. Cambridge: Norfolk, Suffolk and Cambridgeshire Strategic Health Authority.

RAWOrg (2011). *The End of Delivering Race Equality? Perspectives of frontline workers and service-users from racialised groups*. London: RAWORg. www.mind.org.uk/media/273467/the-end-of-delivering-race-equality.pdf (accessed 18 November, 2015).

17

The Sunrise Project: helping adults recover from psychiatric drugs

Terry Simpson

Over 40 years ago, when I was first a mental patient, I escaped from the men's ward and, heavily sedated, wandered into a day room for elderly patients. I sat down in a semi-circle of elders and they stared back at me in silence for what seemed like hours. I was convinced that my life had passed away in the dream of being a mental patient and that I was now old myself, even though I was only 23.

This story now seems symbolic of how disabled I felt taking psychiatric drugs. They never worked well for me. Partly this was because I was forced to have chlorpromazine against my will several times, which felt like a terrible assault. It led to blackouts, amnesia and a general uncomfortable feeling of being strangely divorced from the world around me. During another hospitalisation I was made to take haloperidol, which had the effect of sending muscles in my neck and face into spasm so that my head was twisted violently, my face made grotesque masks, while my teeth ground together as if they'd break. On other occasions the spasms extended to my back so that I was thrown to the floor as if by an invisible wrestler, like the Brad Pitt character in the film Fight Club. Nurses at first thought I was 'acting out' and didn't believe this was the effect of the drug. I think this shows how little the people who administer drugs know about the effects they have.

After my last hospitalisation in 1985, I told my doctor I intended to stop taking psychiatric drugs. He laughed and said I would be ill for the rest of my life, and applauded the fact that I had found a job as a hospital porter – 'You'll be in the right place when you get ill again.' It wasn't encouraging but I stopped taking the drugs anyway. For two weeks I had horrible flu-like symptoms and felt dreadful. Then quite suddenly I felt better, much better than I had since I started taking the drugs. I never took drugs again or went near a mental institution as a patient.

The healing power of listening and being heard

I was lucky enough around that time to find a support group outside the mental health system. The other members were a teacher, a general practitioner (family doctor), and a student about to become a university lecturer, who all had experience of being a patient in a mental health institution. They were an impressive group and at first I felt out of place with these well-dressed, respectable people, but when I listened to their stories I realised that they weren't so different from me, and that we all felt damaged by the experience of being inpatients and taking psychiatric drugs. I'm convinced that, as the months passed, it was this healing space and being heard by my peers, without judgement, that began to heal me. This was my introduction to co-counselling (known also as re-evaluation counselling[1]), and I've continued to use this method to this day. I think that's largely why I've been able to deal with the issues my life has thrown up, and to do successful paid work in and at the edges of the mental health system for the last 25 years. This has included several years of working as a patient advocate in my home city, Leeds, England, and then eight years managing the UK Advocacy Network,[2] a nationwide network of peer-led advocacy organisations that at its peak had over 300 member groups.

Origins of the Sunrise Project

When I first began to get involved in mental health work, I was very influenced by Judi Chamberlin's brilliant account of survivor-led crisis services in the US (Chamberlin, 1978). I was one of the founding members of Leeds Survivor-Led Crisis Service,[3] an attempt to set up something similar in England, which has operated successfully since 1999. The idea of a centre run by 'experts by experience' has always inspired and attracted me, so when co-counsellors began to talk about the idea of a centre to help people get off psychiatric drugs, I was very interested.

---

1. See www.rc.org (accessed 12 November, 2015).

2. See www.u-kan.co.uk (accessed 12 November, 2015).

3. See www.lslcs.org.uk (accessed 12 November, 2015).

Survivors, relatives, and worker allies who use co-counselling have met for many years to support each other to heal from our mental health experiences and think about what a rational system might look like. Janet Foner, a US co-counsellor (who co-founded the radical US group Mindfreedom[4]), wrote a master's thesis on an alternative centre that would use co-counselling (Foner, 1986). When she teamed up with a doctor who practised co-counselling and had decided he no longer felt comfortable prescribing psychiatric drugs for 'mental health problems', things took off and they formed a board to take the idea forward, which I joined.

What is the Sunrise Project?

The key idea behind the Sunrise Project is the use of co-counselling. This is an effective form of peer counselling that involves sharing available time equally between the parties. We think that the aware attention of another human is a key part of our healing, and that all humans have a natural healing process that shows in, for instance, laughing or crying. We think these lead to the release of old, hurtful experiences that are the cause of our minds working in unhelpful ways. The ability to release or discharge feelings involved with painful experiences is not just meaningless 'emoting' but the active ingredient in our healing. Once discharged we can then re-evaluate those old experiences, learning from them and integrating the new knowledge into current life. Both these processes, of discharging and re-evaluating, are impaired by psychiatric drugs, which have the effect of numbing us to our feelings, or creating a state of mind where we are confused and distracted from them.

We would like eventually to have a place, the Sunrise Center,[5] which will be a residential centre where up to six adults will get support while they stop taking psychiatric drugs. Residents will learn co-counselling to resolve their emotional issues. At the present time we think more than 1,000 people have used co-counselling to recover from their experience in the mental health system and over 100 people have used the method to get off and recover from the effects of psychiatric drugs.

On a typical day, residents will have several co-counselling sessions. We may begin with one-way counselling if a person doesn't have enough attention for someone else, but the aim would be for a peer relationship to develop as soon as possible. Paying attention to and thinking about someone else's struggles is a very useful and empowering thing to do, and an important part of the healing process.

---

4. See www.mindfreedom.org/ (accessed 12 November, 2015).

5. www.pvsunrise.org (accessed 12 November, 2015).

As far as possible, staff and residents will interact with each other as peers, not as patients and providers. People will plan their own healing process and proceed at their own pace. There will be time for residents to garden, exercise, create art and partake in other activities that take their attention off the emotional work. It's important to get a balance between dealing with difficult issues and having attention on present time activities.

Residents will work alongside staff on day-to-day activities of cooking, cleaning etc. Everyone will have an equal responsibility for the upkeep of the centre.

Before coming to the centre, residents will be encouraged to form a support team in the community where they live. This will consist of fellow co-counsellors, but also supportive family members and friends. When the person returns home, the support team will continue the work begun at the centre. Former residents and their support teams will remain in touch with people at the centre by phone for follow-up as needed. Support and connection are key issues in coming off psychiatric drugs, and isolation is one of the main reasons people fail. I was lucky to make it, but many people, including friends of mine, try to get off drugs on their own and, if they fail, get disappointed and too frightened to try again.

Challenges

Funding

The main challenge we've faced so far has been a financial one. We have currently raised over $165,000 and think we need about four times that amount to set up the centre and have money on hand for the first year's operating expenses. A danger we intend to avoid is, to get the project going, accepting major funding from a source that requires us to compromise the radical intention of our project. However this means that progress towards our goal has been slow, as we try to raise funds through individual donations and fundraising efforts or look for fund-giving bodies who will allow us to develop without compromising our principles.

So that the work can continue to develop while we are raising the money for an actual centre, we have begun to organise a series of weekend workshops where people can plan, support groups can form and begin to work together, and people on drugs can attend and begin the work. So far (by January 2016) we've had three such workshops. At the moment the intention is to run these every six months, but if more people can be trained to lead them, then they could be more frequent, and in different places.

Producing evidence

What evidence do we have that this process can work? In a later section I've listed some of what we've learned through trial and error about what works to support people stop taking psychiatric drugs. We have not tried to gather information using currently accepted research methods like randomised controlled trials. Nevertheless co-counselling is based on empirical observation, and no new development in technique or practice is accepted until it has been successfully shown to work throughout the network of tens of thousands of people who practise co-counselling worldwide.

Already many people have used co-counselling to help them stop taking psychiatric drugs; some have applied similar methods to those we plan to use at the Sunrise Project. An example from my own experience: I was part of a group of people who helped someone who wanted to stop taking a benzodiazepine, which he had taken for a number of years. He now considers that the group's support was crucial in helping him to stop taking this drug safely. Since he lived in another city, I could only support him through telephone sessions and, since one of his main problems was not sleeping, we generally had these sessions late at night, just before he tried to sleep. In his sessions he addressed his fears about the consequences of not sleeping and possibly getting depressed again. After our sessions he generally slept well and gradually the fear receded. Along with the support he was getting from others, he gained confidence that he would succeed in stopping the drug successfully, and over a period of months tapered down the amount he was taking, and finally stopped altogether.

Why do we think this project is important?

There is a significant body of information that exposes the dangers of all types of psychiatric drugs. Even people who support the use of drugs admit they all have side effects. Research suggests that life expectancy is reduced considerably by the use of such drugs. People talk about the 'risk' of coming off, but staying on them is even more risky for the person. I've personally known several long-term psychiatric drug users who have arguably died prematurely, in their 40s and 50s, including a good friend of mine last year. She didn't drink or smoke, but couldn't control her weight, which had increased greatly since taking psychiatric drugs, and died at the age of 57. She had tried unsuccessfully to stop taking the drugs several times over the decades she had been on them, with virtually no support from within the system to do this.

Most facilities that treat people with 'mental health' issues do so in ways that disempower people, as well as encouraging long-term use of drugs. They may not want to do this, but if one set of people are defined as 'experts' and the others as passive recipients, this is fairly inevitable. Disempowered people, dependent on 'experts' to help them, then become the 'revolving door' patients who are hard to treat successfully, and the system perpetuates itself.

There is a growing number of people who want to stop taking psychiatric drugs and find alternative ways of dealing with strong emotions and past hurts. People need information about how they can do this, and an environment that is conducive to coming off drugs safely. The prevalence of drugs means we haven't explored other ways of healing anything like enough, although there is a growing body of knowledge about how to help people through extreme distress.

What we've learned

We take it as a fundamental principle that it is always the person's own decision to stop using the drugs, not ours or anyone else's.

In general it's good for people who are helping someone to get off psychiatric drugs to have sessions about their own feelings and confusion about drugs, and any hopelessness about the person's ability to succeed, or their own feelings of urgency. Dealing with any issues about our own mental health history and memories relating to the mental health system, or our own experiences related to addictions and drug use of any kind (including alcohol and street drugs), is also useful.

It helps to have a relaxed and confident attitude that the person trying to get off psychiatric drugs can recover completely, and that they can take control of the process and trust their own thinking. We encourage people to work early on memories of being disappointed, having discharge suppressed (being told to stop crying, being angry etc), or early feelings of powerlessness and hopelessness.

Other ways that we've found to be effective are encouraging a person to make the decision to stop using psychiatric drugs, and then to discharge any feelings about this, to work on their own stories about taking drugs (including where they have been part of an ongoing daily routine for a long time), and to consider what did/do they get out of being on drugs, and what they would have to face and discharge if they came off them. We also try to enable people to focus on the present as much as possible, and support them to go after their dreams and set up their lives so they can do that.

Practically it's useful to help a person to set up a large support system of co-counsellors and others who can be called on during the drug withdrawal period. Family members and friends can be taught the basics of co-counselling, including confidentiality and listening, and can be included in the support team. It may be useful for one person to be a 'key' supporter, who'll help make sure the team meets to think about and discharge any feelings of their own. Also it's useful to set up sessions with other allies for mutual support; to learn about drugs and the withdrawal process – particularly drugs the person you are trying to help is taking – and to support the person to make a plan for stopping their use of drugs and keep up to date with how this is going.

The support and help of doctors and other medical staff can be useful. We encourage helpers to stay in good communication with them, and deal with any of their own feelings that might get in the way.

We think that it's not useful for the counsellor to express a moral stance against drugs, to blame or criticise the client for taking drugs, put pressure on him/her or create an atmosphere of urgency.

A different way of doing 'mental health'

The Sunrise Center is incorporated as a 'non-profit' organisation (in England we would call this a charity) and has tax exempt status in the US. We have a board of directors, a fundraising committee, and many people interested in working there, as well as many people waiting to come to the centre as residents.

The board has nine people, mostly in the US, but also from Canada and England (me), who meet through a monthly phone conference. The majority are mental health system survivors, and the rest are relatives of survivors or allies. There's also a regular fundraising call, and a yearly weekend get-together for the board and people on the fundraising team.

We are also running a series of workshops (described in the section 'What we've learned'), where support teams can meet and use the process of co-counselling together, and where the people who want to get off drugs can start the process in a protected environment.

On the Sunrise board meetings we've talked about the centre becoming a training facility where doctors, mental health workers and others can come to learn about the process of coming off psychiatric drugs safely through using the peer counselling techniques of co-counselling. We envisage that, once proven, this example can be replicated, and many other such centres will be set up. Some people have already expressed an interest in this. We hope in the end that the model of healing without drugs, with peer support, will become the norm, and replace a system based on drugs and shock.

One advantage of this way of doing things is its sustainability. Giving people the tools to take control in their own lives again will not only lead to people ending dependency on the mental health system, and the cost implications of this, but they will in turn become a resource for others who are trying to free themselves from psychiatric drugs.

In 'Burnt Norton', the first in TS Eliot's *Four Quartets* (1943), the rose garden is the symbol for the path not (yet) travelled, the alternative reality. Eliot writes: 'What might have been and what has been/Point to one end, which is always present.' It's not too late to have the mental health system of our dreams.

References

Chamberlin J (1978). *On Our Own: patient-controlled alternatives to the mental health system*. New York: Hawthorn Books.

Eliot TS (1943). 'Burnt Norton'. *Four Quartets*. New York: Harcourt, Brace &Co.

Foner J (1986). *An Alternative Non-Residential Mental Health Center*. Master's thesis. Harrisburg, PA: Pennsylvania State University.

WORKING IN PARTNERSHIP

18

More voice, less ventriloquism: building a mental health recovery archive

Dolly Sen and Anna Sexton

This chapter is about how a group of people with lived experience and a professional archivist, together built the Mental Health Recovery Archive:[1] why we did it, how we worked together as co-producers, what worked well and what we found particularly challenging about the process. The project was born from Anna's PhD work exploring participatory approaches to building archives. It was a response to the Wellcome Library's archive and manuscript collections on mental health,[2] which predominantly tell the story from the point of view of the asylum, the medical professional, the psychiatrist and the psychoanalyst. The Wellcome Library collections include case notes that allow us to gaze in at the individual patients in the system, picking up details about pervading views on behaviour and treatment. However what we can see, know and construct about these pasts is heavily filtered through a lens controlled by those with power over the patient. Occasionally there are offerings penned in the hand of the patient, such as letters to family members or pieces of creative work, but these always and only have a place in the case notes because someone other than the patient has decided to put them there.

The Mental Health Recovery Archive aims to show that individuals with lived experience can tell their stories and that these stories are valued and have a permanent space, alongside the stories told by the system, the institution and the medical professional, that is open now to anyone and everyone to explore.

---

1. The Mental Health Recovery Archive is available at http://www.mentalhealthrevoery.omeka.net
2. The other mental health archives are available at http://wellcomelibrary.org

The archive is based around the narratives of Anna Sexton, Dolly Sen, Stuart Baker-Brown, Andrew Voyce and Peter Bullimore. Anna came to the project as an archivist and PhD researcher with an interest in disrupting the power relations that can sit within and around archives. The relationships between Anna, Stuart, Dolly, Peter and Andrew are what built the archive.

This chapter is presented in the form of conversations between Dolly and Anna about the history and inspiration for the archive and the politics and principles that inform it.

I couldn't leave survivor voices in the minority

Dolly: I hadn't worked on an archive before and I didn't really know what it entailed. But I saw it as a new, interesting experience, which is why I agreed to take part. When I heard how little survivor narrative and experience was kept in the mental health archives (only seven per cent found at the beginning of the project), I knew I couldn't leave those voices in the minority.

Archives show who has the power in a given section of society, charting this through history. It's not just the lack of authentic voice; the representation of mental health through, for instance, patients' case notes does not give the person a voice or a life, or tell their truth. It is a bit like lions demonstrating bird song in roars. Why should the hunters give the history of the hunted? Why should the people who've never visited a land be that country's prime historians? How can you arrive at truth when there is such imbalance of power, where there is censorship by omission or invalidation, where our words are seen as sickness? Who gets to speak in history, and who is listened to?

I realised I couldn't complain that the voices of survivors or people who have used mental health services aren't there if I am not willing to speak up myself.

What was valuable about the experience was the telling of my story. I haven't told my story yet in psychiatry. Mental health services read their script, I read my script, and nothing of any deep meaning is ever exchanged. Professionals may know the mountains, their climate, but have they ever climbed them? They might know what goes into the poisoned fruit of medication, but they have never eaten it. They might even know its language, but they will always speak it with an accent, and will lose so much in translation. They record observed data on an unobservable world. They objectify subjective experience and then wonder why there is a clash of mental and emotional cultures. Psychiatry has to rewrite and revise itself. Its story has hurt too many people; it needs to rewrite its script, and stop writing crappy sequels.

Psychiatry is not a mechanism that is able to relieve mental distress. It polices socially sanctioned behaviour, and (among other things) gives the people who go through its system a deep sense of shame that they were sensitive to trauma or the brutalisation of their situation in life. Anna had no such agenda. She wanted to hear my story without bringing shame or pathology into the equation.

Why does it need an archive initiated by somebody who has no mental health training for me to tell my truth? Truth is not sanity, truth is not in my medical notes. Truth is what I was able to tell Anna without it being undermined.

Anna was not an expert in the disempowering sense of the term but she was professional in the sense that she knew about archives. She did what very few professionals do in mental health: she shared her life with me in talking about her family, for example. She also did something that allowed trust and authentic disclosure: she made me the mental health expert and the voice of my story, while offering support and guidance in the archival process. There was nothing to tell me that my guard should go up. From the start it was an open, fluid relationship.

Blank canvas vs realisable venture

Anna: The Mental Health Recovery Archive aims to contest power relations running through the construction of records. It aims to challenge the status quo in relation to who gets to create the types of records that are subsequently held up by society as significant and worthy of ongoing preservation. I will try here to unravel the complexity around the extent to which I feel we achieved these aims.

I believe we pushed some boundaries, but we didn't fully disrupt ingrained power relations. Part of this felt beyond our control – constraints pushing in on us shaped what we could do, and we faced unequal starting positions ingrained within broader societal systems. However, although at times I felt 'powerless' to do anything more than point up the unequal power balance between me and the participants, there were also times when I was perhaps 'powerful' and missed the opportunity to adequately share control. At times I was too quick to close down the doors of joint exploration, as I hurried through the initial stages of the project to turn the blank canvas into a realisable venture. Reflecting back, I can see at least two points in the project with what I will call 'participatory potential', where I could have invited the participants more fully into the process of shaping project outcomes but instead maintained (unnecessary?) boundaries between our roles. The first was in shaping ideas around what the 'archive' should be, and the second was in choosing 'recovery' as the theme for the personal narratives.

As an archivist, I have had a long relationship with this construct called an 'archive'. My professional training taught me to see it from an organisational/ administrative bias. This view has been challenged within my field by a discourse that emphasises that archives can also be sites of 'evidence of me' (McKemmish, 1996) – sites where personal and collective memory can be made and remade. I was therefore keen to explore the 'archive' as personal narrative and I took this vision to the participants. This formed the basis of what we then went on to construct. What if, instead of giving them my vision, I had initiated a two-way conversation? What might an archive reflecting Dolly, Andrew, Peter and Stuart have looked like if instigated from a blanker canvas?

The decision that troubles me most is my suggestion to the participants that we use 'recovery' as the overarching theme for their personal narratives. My degree of influence here is difficult to disentangle. In making the suggestion, I was undoubtedly influenced by the recovery narratives I had read where the term was framed positively as a concept that was being co-constructed by survivors and mental health professionals. I now have a more nuanced perspective on what 'recovery' represents as an ideology and as a system; in fact part of the backlash against recovery has evolved alongside the construction of the Mental Health Recovery Archive. Dolly, Andrew, Stuart and Peter recognised its potential to carry and give hope but they also recognised the potential for it to be used as a form of control.

We agreed collectively that their narratives would be critically reflective about the concept of 'recovery', questioning it and challenging the way it is used (and abused) by the mental health system. That critical reflection is apparent when reading the narratives, but I am now aware that in using the frame 'recovery' we have potentially alienated those who have painful associations with the term because of the ways in which it has been applied in mental health service provision. My regret is missing the opportunity to leave the frame of the archive open, as something that would emerge *through* Dolly, Peter, Andrew and Stuart's narratives. I wanted to get something solid in place for us to work around and in, but if I could go back to the beginning I wouldn't be so afraid of openness and a seeming lack of structure in the early phases of the project. I would go with fluidity and trust that the doors would open without being forced. It has been a steep learning curve for me, and I will take what I've learned into future participatory work.

Part of the complexity in seeking to take a participatory approach to constructing an archive is the rhetoric around transformative participation. I have wanted to foster relational working that enables co-construction and a shared authority. The threads of power and control running through this type of work are a far more complex entanglement than simplistic mantras of 'give your control away' suggest. Co-construction can never erase all the differences between us but it does need to start by acknowledging those differences, whether they are in expertise, experience, degrees of influence or access to resources, and to recognise that the holder of expertise and influence will vary, depending on the context. It is about using these differences positively as constructive forces where possible, while also recognising that at times the imbalances are negatives that should be challenged and transformed through the co-working process. Discerning when an imbalance is negative rather than positive and then attempting to redress the power dynamic is a difficult process. In part I think success depends on the strength of the underpinning relationships between the participants.

One area of imbalance that needs to be acknowledged relates to the gulf in access to resources. As the PhD researcher, I came into the project with a bursary from the Arts and Humanities Research Board; the expectation was that Dolly, Andrew, Stuart, and Peter should give their expertise with no payment other than to cover expenses. This is in itself deeply unfair. However this material divide on access to resources continues beyond the construction of the Mental Health Recovery Archive, into our dissemination activities. I have been able to access academic funds to travel internationally to deliver conference papers about the archive, but there is no funding to take ANY participants as co-presenters. This problem is bigger and more systemic than the Mental Health Recovery Archive. If academia wants to take participatory research seriously, then these differences need to be addressed and those of us who sit on the inside of academia need to be vocal about the need for change.

What does it mean to work in partnership?

Dolly: It was a true partnership because it was two people coming together with different expertise to create something dynamic, new and unique.

Anna and I shared a professional relationship but there were not the boundaries that are evident in relationships with mental health professionals, which are governed by risk assessments and you have to guard against personal connection. Anna didn't have that baggage; she saw me as her equal. I didn't censor myself with Anna, she had the whole of me, not some human being barely perceptible behind a label, which is how some clinicians see you.

The difference it made to work with someone with little preconception as to how to work with survivors except to come to it from a position of empathy and intelligence was so palpable, I see that as a necessary precondition. Her approach was to ask, 'What works for you? How shall we work when things get difficult?'

Twenty-five years in the mental health system and this is still one of the first times that someone has asked me about my story. When you are in that relationship with a doctor or a psychiatric nurse, they already have their own idea of what your distress is about. They don't ask you to know you; they look for the symptoms in their little book and that is how they make sense of your world and your distress. I think it would be more powerful if they asked us, 'What has made you distressed now? Is there something that has made you the way you are today?' And that would give us a chance to say, 'Actually yes, I know what has caused my distress, to me it is very obvious.' Why couldn't I say that in psychiatry or the mental health system? Why does it have to be an archivist, with no clinical experience, who asks that question? I saw the archive as a place for creative expression but I also saw it in a political context as well, as a challenge to the system that demanded, 'Why aren't you doing this? Why haven't you done this for me?'

My criticism of services wasn't seen as a personality disorder; my fear and mistrust of society's perception of mental distress wasn't paranoia; my sadness wasn't a sign of depression; my anger wasn't a sign of schizophrenia; my joy was not a sign of mania. The emotions were seen as human and an appropriate response to experiences. The only expectation this non-medical non-survivor had of me was to be a human. There were no symptoms, only difficulties to be discussed and negotiated and, usually, handled with compassion. My words and experience were meaningful to Anna. What made it feel like a genuine partnership was that we shared in the proper sense of the word: ideas, thoughts, experiences, emotions, fun and work.

There was some imbalance of control. Anna got a bursary to work on her PhD; we got expenses. She framed the archive into being about recovery. So we didn't have complete choice in what the archive should be about; this was due to time constraints on all sides. But whatever the subject is, we can position ourselves to tell our truth.

The crux of why I did it is that in 100 years' time people won't get a whitewashed version of what it is like to be someone like me. They will get a truthful account, one that has both criticism and also hope. That was quite a hard balancing act. I want my story to be one of many that says why the current mental health system needs to change. A voice and story without equality is an act of ventriloquism that can never be as beautiful as one with.

Anna: In working on the Mental Health Recovery Archive I had the privilege to get to know four people who I feel I have shared (in different ways) a genuine connection with. I really like Dolly, Stuart, Andrew and Peter and I felt their warmth and acceptance from the very start. At times we worked collectively, particularly when we were gearing up to launch the archive, but I also got to spend time with them individually, and establishing one-to-one relationships was a vital part of the process.

From the start I have been aware that I am asking Dolly, Andrew, Stuart and Peter to publish their personal narratives in the online archive for all to see; I don't take that lightly. If I am expecting them to share their lives and history with me and with others, then it cannot possibly be an equal process unless I am willing to open myself up in a similar way, both to them and to others. I have deliberately pushed at the professional/personal boundary in this project. In my relationship with each of the participants, little by little I have been open about my past and present, everything that shapes who I am. Of course relationships take time to develop; the openness has grown in response to the unfolding dynamic of trust between us – something that has been carefully weighed up and not naively assumed. I believe that my distance from the mental health system has enabled me to take this approach.

As well as opening up individually to the four participants, I took what I see as the more difficult decision to make myself, and aspects of my personal history, visible within the archive in a section where I talk about myself. I describe what has led me to want to be involved in the construction of the archive and aspects of my personal story that have an impact and a bearing in this context. This is because, first, I wanted to embed myself in the archive so that those who come to browse through Dolly, Andrew, Stuart and Peter's stories can make an informed judgement about the degree to which it really is (as it set out to be) their story on their own terms, and the degree to which I am present as a co-constructer and shaper of the archive.

Second, I have sought to make myself visible because I needed to experience something of what it is like to open yourself up to the public gaze, to make yourself vulnerable to the judgements of others on personal aspects of your story. If I expect Dolly, Andrew, Peter and Stuart to do this then I should be prepared to go through the same. I found it an uncomfortable and unsettling process and it taught me a great deal about the costs of making your personal history public from a contributor's perspective. It has reinforced and underscored the deep respect I have for Dolly, Andrew, Peter and Stuart, who continually put themselves and their experiences out there in differing forms. I hope that in a small way what we have created in the Mental Health Recovery Archive can add to the momentum for transformation across archives and mental health. In both contexts the stories of individuals with lived experience need to be heard in ways that ensure they are the ones who shape the representations of themselves.

Possibilities in survivor/non-survivor research

In many ways the 'survivor'/'non-survivor' distinction between us was useful and constructive in enabling co-productive research. It meant that Dolly and the other participants were entirely and rightly the experts both in relation to their own experience and in relation to mental health contexts more broadly. The participants have shaped what Anna has learnt about mental health; she came with very little prior knowledge. The psychiatric labels that the participants carried were only vaguely familiar to her and she decided to only read survivor-initiated (or co-produced) literature alongside listening to Peter, Dolly, Andrew and Stuart to shape her understandings. Having not experienced anything similar, and being unconnected to the mental health system, meant that Dolly and the participants necessarily acted as Anna's guides.

The 'survivor'/'non-survivor' distinction became more palpable, and for Anna more uncomfortable, during the dissemination phase of the project, at the launch and at conferences and meetings, particularly where survivors have been assessing the validity of the archive from their perspectives. Anna's impression is that legitimacy for 'survivor'/'non-survivor' collaborations is (understandably) not easily given. The starting point feels like it is, 'What right have you as a non-survivor to encroach on this ground?' Although it made Anna feel uncomfortable, that question is valid and important; trust has to be earned and it is particularly difficult for it to develop when there is the weight of past injustices and power imbalances. Imbalances which continue to inform the present.

Opening the archive up for comment from archivists, survivors, non-survivors and others has been a useful process. Most reactions from survivors have been positive. Some comments and questions have prompted us to critically reflect back on the archive. Some have voiced concerns that removing an individual's story from the collective history of the survivor movement is a weakness of the project and is potentially disempowering for the survivor movement itself. This raises questions around whether it is legitimate to take a life history approach that is individualistic, rather than collective, in its starting point. While it is vital to be aware and wary of the potential for the archive to disempower, our justification is that all starting points have strengths and weaknesses: in a collective there is a danger that the individual is lost; with an individual approach there is a danger that the collective (and its power) is dissolved. It seems that perhaps both are necessary and legitimate approaches that answer different needs.

Should survivors only undertake survivor history and survivor research? This issue is reminiscent of the broader debates within the archives field around independent grassroots community archives, which often grow in response to marginalisation and gaps in the records held by mainstream archival institutions (Gilliland & Flinn, 2013). Some community archivists opt to maintain and defend their boundaries: their power and legitimacy is gained from their distance from the mainstream. Others seek out collaborative relationships, sharing expertise and resources. This is most successful when a genuine 'shared authority' is sought on both sides, with the community having the right to contribute to steering the archive in relation to issues such as its development, preservation and access. Rather than labelling one approach as 'right' and one approach as 'wrong', it is perhaps more helpful to evaluate each approach in terms of its opportunities and threats. Critically reflecting on these is part and parcel of the process of history making.

References

Gilliland A, Flinn A (2013). *Community Archives: what are we really talking about?* Keynote address at 'Nexus, Confluence, and Difference: Community Archives meets Community Informatics', the CIRN Community Informatics Conference 2013, 28–30 October, in Prato, Italy. Available at: http://www.ccnr.infotech.monash.edu.au/assets/docs/prato2013_papers/gilliland_flinn_keynote.pdf (accessed 12 November, 2015).

McKemmish S (1996). Evidence of me. *Archives & Manuscripts 24*(1): 28–45.

19

Teaching (like) crazy in a mad-positive school: exploring the charms of recursion

Danielle Landry and Kathryn Church

> *Teaching in the social sciences in universities is a political act. This is not a matter of the expression of specific political values; it is built into the theories and methodologies of every social science. (Smith, 2006: 25)*

We are sitting together at the small round table in Kathryn's office. Winter darkness seeps in from an east-facing window but the room is warm, full of colour and bursting with piles of paper. Seizing a late afternoon lull in demand, we turn our attention to the prospect of searching for a rose garden. The moment is somewhat fraught. As our first venture into co-authorship, this chapter is definitely cause for reflection on entry points and locations. Kathryn is Director of the School of Disability Studies at Ryerson University and a tenured faculty member. Danielle is an instructor and research assistant in the school and, as such, much more precariously situated in terms of her labour. Kathryn's involvement as a mad movement ally dates back 30 years to the first formations of 'consumer participation' (Church, 1993; Church & Reville, 2012). Danielle's engagement in the mad movement is more recent, more direct in terms of her identifications, and more diverse across sites of scholarly activism (Costa et al, 2012). Thus, differentially, we are steeped in the complexities of producing alternatives to psychiatric knowledge.

We have worked together for almost a decade. Much of what we know in relation to each other is derived from using Disability Studies as an intellectual and organisational base for generating what we speak of, increasingly, as Mad Studies[1] (LeFrançois, Menzies & Reaume, 2013; Church, 2015). The programme at Ryerson University is 15 years old. It has three full-time faculty members, a shifting roster of part-time instructors, and a relatively small budget. Grappling with disabling social relations rather than individual impairment is a defining characteristic of the curriculum. Using online and on-site modalities, we deliver courses year round to students all over Ontario. Offerings include an online course[2] titled 'Mad People's History', for which Danielle is now the instructor (Reville, 2013), and an in-person course, 'A History of Madness', which is taught as an upper-level Liberal Arts elective. Between the two, we reach approximately 400 students a year with counter-hegemonic interpretations of 'mental illness'.

Charmed by recursion

As evening approaches, our conversation meanders in and around the complexities of doing this work. As we talk, we are struck by the resonances that some activities have with each other – primarily, the ease of teaching Mad Studies courses within a School of Disability Studies that is connected to Toronto's mad community. The school offers its space to mad community groups for meetings, supports symposiums, festivals, talks and other mad community events, creates academic pathways for mad students, and then supports their achievements and fosters critical scholarship. Not surprisingly, several staff members and students in Disability Studies identify as members of the mad community. None of this is consciously co-ordinated but it all fits together.

We are further struck – even thunderstruck – by the exact opposite in terms of our broader interventions: in the neoliberal university, the mental health system, and with the public. We feel it when we are asked to share our thoughts on the 'crisis of student mental health' over lunch with well-meaning academics. Silently glancing at one another, we wonder which of us is willing to do the work this time? We feel it when a student-led taskforce collects 'mental wellness' survey data and asks students to 'share their stories' for the final report. Or when we are made to repeat our position at each and every meeting of the campus-wide mental health taskforce because someone new has arrived and does

---

1. We locate Mad Studies as a radical, inter-disciplinary 'project of inquiry, knowledge production and political action' that draws from people 'whose lives have collided with the powers of institutional psychiatry' to critique and transcend 'psy-centred ways of thinking, behaving, relating and being'. Particularly important to us is Mad Studies as critical pedagogy against discrimination and oppression that is *nested* (our emphasis) 'in the immediate practicalities of everyday human struggle' (LeFrançois, Menzies & Reaume, 2013: 15–17).

2. With online courses, all learning is done in a virtual environment using computers and an internet connection.

not understand why we keep using the word 'mad' – yet no one ever asks the psychology professor or the human resources rep to justify their use of the term 'mental illness'. At times, we get fired up, hopeful that we can make change on campus. But often we are left disheartened when we do make the effort but are not being heard, or only a handful of people turn up.

Danielle feels these moments when she is asked to participate in service system-organised client feedback events, knowing full well that the event is simply ticking a box on someone's list; what is proposed will move ahead as planned, regardless of her input. Or when service users are asked to attend day-long 'community consultations' involving mental health professionals but, magically, all of the men in suits vanish before lunch. Even when participating in survivor-driven conferences within the mental health sector, it's noticeable that, despite invitations, few non-survivor mental health workers or facility staff bother to attend. The bumps, bruises and breaks of these encounters, the awkward silences and outright refusals register with us deeply – individually and collectively. How can we frame these observations in ways that are theoretically fruitful?

Energies rising, we plunder the nearby bookshelves for a well-worn Canadian text on social movements and social research (Frampton et al, 2006). From the chapter on 'political activist/s as ethnographers' we tease out George Smith's use of the term 'recursion' to explore 'how the everyday experiences of people can have the same social form as the experiences of others, at other times and places' (p36) and, more specifically, how texts are used to hold the same forms of ruling in place across sites. Not only does the term illuminate the ways in which psychiatry achieves global reach and local saturation (Mills & Fernando, 2014), it also gives us another way to name and think about the turbulence of making Mad Studies. The alternative speech and practices we are using 'bump up' against the textually mediated productions of 'mental health' reproduced more generally within the university.

Our understanding is further enlivened when we trace Smith's reference to the work of mathematician Douglas Hofstadter, whose 'eternal golden braiding' of Kurt Godel, MC Escher and JS Bach won him a Pulitzer Prize. In a beautifully lucid paragraph he describes recursion as:

> … *nesting and variations on nesting. The concept is very general.*
> *(Stories inside stories, movies inside movies, paintings inside paintings,*
> *Russian dolls inside Russian dolls (even parenthetical comments*
> *inside parenthetical comments!) – these are just a few of the charms of*
> *recursion) (Hofstadter, 1979: 127 – our emphasis).*

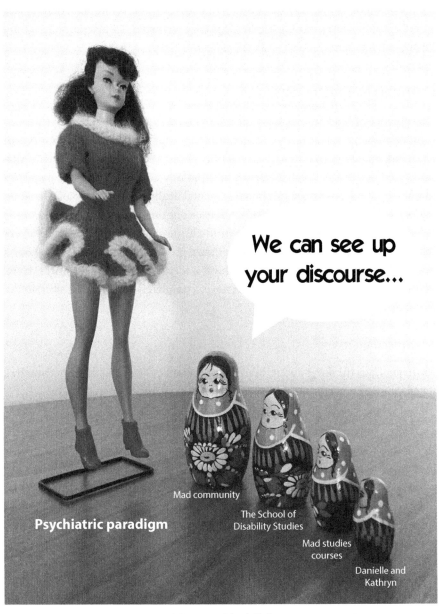

Playing with dolls[3]
© Danielle Landry

---

3. Our thanks to Jenna Reid for sparking the remark in the speech bubble

Nesting and variations on nesting! Now *here* is a notion we like – not just to tag the 'booted out of the nest' discomfort that arises when dominant social forms spiral into our work, but for the fierce joy we feel when things *do* fit, hold and enlarge each other.

Learning to teach crazy

Our practice of Mad Studies is comprised of many kinds of pedagogical occasions – mundane and extraordinary, in and outside the university. One significant landmark is the international dialogue titled 'Mad-Positive in the Academy' that we hosted in 2012. It created a space for scholarly activists from four countries to pursue a mad-positive standpoint on mental health services, formal education and social movements.[4] But when it comes right down to it, our core labour is to engage flesh-and-blood students in institutionally-structured processes of teaching and learning. 'Teaching (like) crazy' gives this traditional endeavour a new political twist: it is a fresh problematic and emergent set of practices. Here, dialogue is a potent tool but one that never completely resolves the situation of the mad-identified partner.

A partner dialogue

Kathryn: I am thinking about 'Mad People's History' and the dilemma you had when you took over as course instructor in 2014. What happened there?

Danielle: As you know, the course that David Reville developed works against the dominant psychiatric paradigm by placing the perspective of mad people at the centre of knowledge formation. It distinguishes between the history of psychiatry as the dominant way of knowing about madness over time, and the history of madness as the suppressed and subordinated knowing of mad people themselves. Echoing the significance of survivor narratives to mad knowledge, David embedded his own narrative in the course. Multimedia teaching tools, such as photographs and web docs, or short documentary films, retain his image. In a multitude of ways, he is indelibly inscribed in the materials.

Kathryn: How intimidating! As programme director, I certainly thought about

---

4. In addition to Disability Studies at Ryerson, the innovative projects we drew from included Comensus (University of Central Lancashire, England), Oor Mad History (a mental health advocacy collective in Edinburgh, Scotland) and the Field School in Social Research, Centre to Study Recovery in Social Contexts, (Columbia University, New York).

the challenges involved in 'course transition'. But perhaps I was not as aware as I should have been about what that process would be like for you – ironic, since I have taught with David and know about his indelibility! I wanted an instructor who was mad identified as well as familiar with this particular course and its history. More than that, I wanted someone who understood how the course was nested within Disability Studies, our particular school and its connections to the mad community. Not an easy combination to find. From our work on other projects, I knew that you had all of the right markings, even if you were not quite there with the formal credentials.

Danielle: In four years of working with David, I had made the course accessible, co-designed workshops, and curated the art exhibits we generated from student work. But I had never taught a course before and was still a graduate student myself. David, however, anticipating his retirement, had prepared me for taking over the course. In fact he did much more than that: he took me to meet with local politicians, to consumer/survivor/ex-patient (c/s/x) organisation meetings, to community gatherings. He gave me opportunities to hone my skills by giving guest lectures in the classroom and the community. Through this process he instilled in me the importance of mentorship. My shift to instructor reflects a conscious commitment by David and the school to create valuable teaching opportunities for young mad scholars – by this I mean not simply people with lived experience but politicised mad instructors applying a critical approach in their teaching practices.

Kathryn: It strikes me as important that you and I share this particular informal training. David mentored me, too, in very similar ways; for several years I walked along with him among the people, places and activities that constituted his world as a politician and an organiser. That is how I learned 'survivor politics' and I drew the same conclusion you did: that it was important for me to bring others along in similar ways. I have never characterised what he did as a partnership development strategy, but it certainly underpins our capacity – yours and mine – to work across difference. With a bit of administrative power, I can now give organisational priority to the kinds of hiring you describe – and that you represent. It has become part of my work to try to open up pedagogical spaces like that, although it might not have become so obvious without those 'walk-alongs'!

Danielle: A further dilemma is that, as a member of the mad community, I feel accountable to accurately represent what is an ongoing activist social history.

However I am uncomfortable with being looked to as a voice of 'authority' on the local history of the c/s/x movement. Learning about the mad movement gave me the opportunity to politicise my own experiences of the psychiatric system as a youth and young adult. Becoming involved in the community has helped to shape my political identity. Nonetheless, I would in no way consider myself an expert in this area; I continue to look to leaders in the movement for knowledge and guidance. University instructors are meant to be experts in their fields, whereas I cannot embrace this notion. The students in my class are adult learners; they come into the classroom full of knowledge and experience. I too am a student in another role, so I recognise myself both as a learner among learners and a teacher among teachers. Expertise then, is not about knowing the facts but about knowing where you are.

Kathryn: I have struggled with authority questions as well, mostly as a working-class woman from small-town western Canada. And I have written about the ones that have troubled my academic practice: for example, the strangeness of doing doctoral research that analysed the use of psychiatric survivor narratives in/against mental health policy formation – but not teaching what I know in favor of people with direct experience (Church, 2013). As an 'outsider' to the mad movement, I have often felt… perhaps, quieted… conscious that others with more of a stake should speak, and wondering how to contribute what I know without silencing or appropriating or professionalising. In order to get tenure, I had to assert a claim to expertise that was more individual than collective when – then and now – I look to movement leaders the same way you do. We are right to do so, I think. But, as you point out, such a stance means challenging conventional academic notions of 'what counts as knowledge' and 'who counts as a knower' – questions that I have situated at the heart of my research methodology course.

Unexpectedly, taking on the director job has helped; the title confers authority, whether I want it or not. Then the issue is how to 'live' that power as it plays against my personal material, and whether it can be used for social justice during the current crisis of neoliberal restructuring. Not a promising scenario but certainly an opportunity to nuance my understanding of authority and expertise: working 'up' the organisational hierarchy as well as working 'down'.

Danielle: In the classroom I have chosen to openly identify as mad from day one because roles concern functions, whereas identity denotes investments (Britzman, 1991). Sharing my identity with students is my way of letting them know that I am invested in bringing about social change for this community.

Teaching an online course can feel disembodied; even more so, I would argue, when you are entrusted with another (mad) person's narrative. As mentioned previously, the course is taught from an insider's perspective, but not my own. At times I feel like the '(wo)man behind the curtain' in *The Wizard of Oz*, as David's narrative remains central to how students move through the curriculum. Students constantly dialogue with me, but they learn through David's narrative, so I need to make my presence known from the outset of the course. My brief experience as an instructor has also taught me about the embodied advantages in the disembodied nature of teaching online – a phenomenon not mentioned in the academic literature. For instance, as a mad instructor I find it beneficial to be able to work from bed or at all hours of the night; I simply log into the course from a laptop. Likewise, I appreciate not having to worry about getting behind on the days when I find I cannot leave the house. In fact, these usually make for my most productive days in the course.

Kathryn: You are at the cutting edge of that discussion, for sure. I truly believe that, as you teach, your own narrative will emerge in dialogue with David's and we will have a new, stronger iteration of the course. I cannot do this 'insider' work. I can only recognise its profound value and stand with you as you do it. I can listen and problem solve along the way, and learn from what you do in ways that extend the knowledge to others so that we build and radiate a strong mad-positive culture. Lately, though, I have had occasion to remember the importance of continuing to identify as an ally, as a mad-positive person who works in alliance, if only because many of our students are in this position across a range of communities. Being an ally is also an active terrain of knowing and learning; it has a politics. I can keep working on that piece of the puzzle but much of 'teaching (like) crazy' still rests with you. (Short pause.) Well, we have opened up some areas here that are quite subtle and could use further discussion. From your perspective, what have we left dangling?

Danielle: Throughout my first term teaching 'Mad People's History', students started coming out as mad. This is not entirely surprising, given the course opens up conversations of madness and, perhaps for the first time, students encounter self-identified and proud mad people acting as powerful pedagogues. Students are encouraged to draw from their own experiences as they move through the course, so some may come to relate to the materials on a personal level, politicising any experiences they may have had with the mental health or psychiatric system. The online classroom also provides a thin veil of invisibility, so coming out, even in small or less public ways, may be more inviting. Clearly something is shifting in terms of people's willingness to open up about their mental health histories, and/ or word has gotten out that this course constitutes a safe space in which to speak from experience. The key piece, I believe, is that this is one of those rare academic spaces where mad people take centre stage (and hold the microphone).

Matthews (2009) uses the Disability Discrimination Act (DDA)[5] as a starting point to discuss how legislation is implemented in the classroom to accommodate the needs of students with invisible disabilities. She argues universities should focus less on identifying and accommodating disabled students based on medical labels; instead they should adopt policies based on the social model of disability and implement a diversity of accessible teaching practices. University policies adapted from these pieces of legislation frequently place the onus on students to come forward, identify as disabled, present medical documentation and articulate their needs to each professor in order to be accommodated. However these policies are premised on a problematic 'common-sense' assumption (Cadwallader, 2010): that all students are able-bodied unless proven otherwise.

Professors, particularly if teaching online, are unlikely to be aware of a student's disability if they choose not to disclose. Opening up conversations about disability/madness may make it easier for students to contact instructors about their specific needs. However some may not feel comfortable disclosing, at first or at all, or they may encounter difficulties in obtaining medical documentation from the required gatekeepers, especially students with invisible disabilities, who are less likely to be believed. To ensure my practices are as mad positive as possible, I have tried to invert the sanist assumptions at play in accommodation policies – to assume instead that everyone is mad until stated otherwise. This means giving students as much time as possible for assignments, checking in with students who 'disappear'/go off the radar, incorporating other forms of accessible media, such as audio recordings and videos to break up the overload of reading, and educating the class on available alternative supports, such as peer support and advocacy groups. Burstow (2003) offers suggestions for making classrooms more accessible to psychiatric survivors, such as taking frequent breaks, accommodating sporadic attendance, and providing food. Many of them do not apply to the online environment; yet adjustments like taking a relaxed pace and making computers and computer literacy programmes available to survivors could be adopted.

---

5. The DDA is somewhat similar to the 2005 Accessibility for Ontarians with Disabilities Act (AODA) but applies nationwide across Canada.

Rippling out

In this chapter we have situated 'teaching (like) crazy' within our exploration of 'the charms of recursion' that characterise a mad-positive school. Using different voices and writing styles, we have tried to sense the vibes, echoes, and concentric circles of partner relations that nurture this emergent practice. Like Freire (1970), we believe that revolutionary change requires education to become the practice of freedom. If we are to foster psychiatric survivor-led alternatives, we must become increasingly skilled in teaching students – in Disability Studies and other disciplines – to think critically about 'mad matters' (LeFrançois, Menzies & Reaume, 2013).

References

Britzman DP (1991). *Practice Makes Practice: a critical study of learning to teach.* Albany, NY: State University of New York Press.

Burstow B (2003). From pills to praxis: psychiatric survivors and adult education. *The Canadian Journal for the Study of Adult Education 17*(1): 1-18.

Cadwallader JR (2010). Stirring up the sediment: the corporeal pedagogies of disabilities. *Discourse: Studies in the Cultural Politics of Education 31*(4): 513–526.

Church K (1993). *Breaking Down/Breaking Through: multi-voiced narratives on psychiatric survivor participation in Ontario's community mental health system.* Unpublished doctoral dissertation. Toronto, ON: Ontario Institute for Studies in Education.

Church K (2013). Making madness matter in academic practice. In: LeFrançois BA, Menzies R, Reaume G (eds) (2013). *Mad Matters: a critical reader in Canadian mad studies.* Toronto: Canadian Scholars' Press (pp181–194).

Church K (2015). 'It's complicated': blending disability and mad studies in the corporatising university. In: Spandler H, Anderson J, Sapey B (eds). *Madness, Distress and the Politics of Disablement.* Bristol: Policy Press (pp261–270).

Church K, Reville D (2012). Mad activism enters its fifth decade: psychiatric survivor organizing in Toronto. In: Choudry A, Hanley J, Shragge E (eds). *Organize!: building from the local for global justice.* Oakland, CA: PM Press (pp189–201).

Costa L, MacFarlane B, Landry D, Voronka J, Reid J, Reville D, Church K (2012). Recovering our stories: a small act of resistance. *Studies in Social Justice 6*(1): 85–101.

Frampton C, Kinsman G, Thompson AK, Tilleczek K (eds) (2006). *Sociology for Changing the World: social movements/social research.* Halifax, NS: Fernwood Publishing.

Freire P (1970). *Pedagogy of the Oppressed.* New York: The Seabury Press.

Hofstadter DR (1979). *Godel, Escher, Bach: an eternal golden braid.* New York: Random House.

LeFrançois BA, Menzies R, Reaume G (eds) (2013). *Mad matters: a critical reader in Canadian mad studies.* Toronto: Canadian Scholars' Press.

Matthews N (2009). Teaching the 'invisible' disabled students in the classroom: disclosure, inclusion and the social model of disability. *Teaching in Higher Education 14*(3): 229–239.

Mills C, Fernando S (2014). Globalizing mental health or pathologizing the Global South? Mapping the ethics, theory and practice of global mental health. *Disability and the Global South: an International Journal 1*(2): 188–202.

Reville D (2013). Is mad studies emerging as a new field of inquiry? In: LeFrancois BA, Menzies R, Reaume G (eds) (2013). *Mad Matters: a critical reader in Canadian mad studies.* Toronto: Canadian Scholars' Press (pp170–180).

Smith DE (2006). George Smith, political activist as ethnographer and sociology for people. In: Frampton C, Kinsman G, Thompson AK, Tilleczek K (eds). *Sociology for Changing the World: social movements/social research.* Halifax, NS: Fernwood Publishing (pp18–26).

Bibliography

The following sources also informed our chapter, although they are not directly cited in the text.

Deroy X, Clegg S (2015). Back in the USSR: introducing recursive contingency into institutional theory. *Organizational Studies 36*(1): 73–90.

Reid J, Poole J (2013). Mad students in the social work classroom? Notes from the beginnings of an inquiry. *Journal of Progressive Human Services 24*(3): 209–222.

Smith GW (1990). Political activist as ethnographer. *Social Problems 37*(4): 629–648.

Smith GW, Mykhalovskiy E, Weatherbee D (2006). A research proposal. In: Smith DE (ed). *Institutional Ethnography as Practice.* Lanham, MD: Rowman & Littlefield Publishers Inc (pp165–180).

20

Peer workers in the mental health system: a transformative or collusive experiment?

Celia Brown and Peter Stastny

This chapter is based on the authors' experiences between 1990 and 1994 while working for a research demonstration project to assess the impact of hiring peer workers ('specialists') to work on Intensive Case Management (ICM) teams in the Bronx. The study showed that the ICM teams with peer specialists had a positive impact on clients' quality of life in several areas, in comparison with teams with paraprofessional workers and those with no additional staff (Felton et al, 1995). Two years after the completion of this project, the New York State Civil Service Commission approved the new job title of 'Peer Specialist' – the first state to do so in the US. Celia Brown was one of the first persons to be hired in New York State as a peer specialist and later became Project Facilitator, where she supervised the peer specialists and interfaced with the ICM programme.

Initially, we conceived of these peer specialists as change agents who would promote positive developments in the way folks were being treated. Was this a reasonable expectation? Nearly 25 years later, the international movement to employ former psychiatric patients or survivors of the mental health system to work within psychiatric services has grown exponentially (Repper & Carter, 2011; Davidson et al, 2012; Stastny & Brown, 2013; Lloyd-Evans et al, 2014). As two of the pioneers of this development, we here reflect on this early experience and provide some thoughts for the future. Our study remains one of the few that shows ex-patients can have an impact on the quality of life of their peers by virtue of their personal experiences (Felton et al, 1996), but whether they can have an impact beyond this narrow focus is hard to ascertain.

Co-optation is an issue

The perspective of Celia Brown, one of the first peer specialists to be employed in New York State.

My experience as a psychiatric survivor guided me in my work as a peer specialist. My skills in practising self-help, peer counselling and in the principles associated with the consumer/survivor movement prepared me to work on the Peer Specialist Project. I was going back to a place where I had been a patient. This time around I became employed in the ICM programme. It was a process to transition from receiving monthly disability benefits to full-time employment. I felt good about working with ICM professionals and felt I could learn from them. But the team didn't embrace me or the other peer specialists as I expected, and it felt as if I was being treated like a mental patient again. I wasn't expecting to have to deal with stigmatising attitudes from the ICM workers. Their concerns were, 'Do we treat the peer specialists like our clients? Will we be their therapists? What do we do if they decompensate?' Initially the peer specialists were excluded from staff meetings where the clients' clinical issues would be discussed. I wanted them to view me as a peer, as a colleague sharing my expertise. The fact that I was an ex-patient in recovery was a challenge for them. This was a powerful indication that the status quo was changing. Our mission was to be role models and change agents for the ICM programme, its clients and the wider system. The ICM programme's purpose was to help clients negotiate services and resources to meet their needs, and thereby establish themselves in the community, avoid rehospitalisations, and build on their strengths. How would ICMs work with us as colleagues? How would they reconcile their preconceived notions and expectations and come to believe that clients' psychiatric diagnoses don't determine whether they can have a meaningful life?

It was a long process, but we made a difference with the ICMs. I was able to explain Medicaid and Social Security benefits from firsthand experience. I understood the system and was able to share my knowledge to assist them with the clients. Initially our role as peer specialists was to participate in the team process, assist in planning and implementing treatment plans, facilitate self-help activities, and establish peer networks and natural supports. Our role was later defined more clearly as aiming to develop our own peer relationships. Consequently, we paired up with several ICM clients with whom we wanted to work. Peer specialists developed a non-medical approach and explored community resources such as recreation, the library and employment opportunities. The purpose of focusing on non-medical approaches is to show people that clients are not just clients; we are people, human beings. You don't have to just be a mental patient. You have the right to be in the community and be an active citizen. Some of the ICMs thought that going to the movies was just a trip and part of the treatment but it was more than that. It taught people about resources in their local community, how to budget their money so they could go out on their own, and got them accustomed to the idea of socialising with friends and family so they wouldn't have to depend on us or the ICMs in the future. I developed peer support relationships; we were like friends in a way. I could step out of this role and help them if needed and they could support me. Peer support was reciprocal.

I realised that in order to effect system change, I would have to keep myself informed about the consumer/survivor/ex-patient movement, and get support from my fellow peer specialists and the project team.

The peer specialist project was successful because it enabled us to bring our own experiences of recovery to the table. The project showed that recovery is possible. Since then, the role of peer specialists has gone through a transformation. The unique expertise of peer specialists working in the system isn't always being used to the fullest extent. The current role of peer specialists needs to be developed according to these key principles: create job descriptions that value our expertise; incorporate peer specialist competencies such as mental health and substance use, psychiatric survivor perspectives, forensic background, homelessness, employment etc.

Co-optation is an issue for peer specialists working in mental health services teams. Inadequate planning and implementation can lead to a misunderstanding of the peer specialist role, and this contributes to peers being co-opted. It's not that all peer specialists are co-opted into the structure of the system; some peers hold fast to their values of recovery and the principles of the consumer/survivor/ex-patient movement. However, when faced with the realities of poverty, homelessness and the need to feed their family, some peer specialists can succumb to co-optation and the pressures of working in the mental health service system.

If I were making changes today in terms of peer specialists working and getting hired, I would ensure that peer support is implemented, emphasise that people can recover, teach people to advocate for themselves, and never forget the triumphs and struggles of their own journey in recovery. I would hire peer supervisors, and build a team of like-minded professionals who really believe in recovery and don't just pay lip service to it. I would create different teams of peer expertise, including peers who are also parents. However, I also believe that the team approach isn't the only way to support people; individual peer support has also proven to be effective.

I've been involved in the survivor movement for many years. The values of the independent movement to fight for human rights and self-determination inform my work. The movement pushes the system to focus on rights. Mental health care should be a choice but often people diagnosed with a mental illness are viewed as incapable of making treatment decisions and can easily lose their rights under current mental health laws.

Peer-run programmes are an important part of supporting peer specialists. Through such programmes, peer specialists can refer people to housing, peer advocacy and trauma-informed training etc. Peer-run programmes help traditional psychiatric staff view these services in a positive way. I think we need peer-run programmes where people can go to access their services. However, it's hard to rely solely on peer-run programmes when there are so few of them or they are integrated in traditional mental health programmes.

I would like the next generation of peer workers to know that their role is to change the system, change the way peers are viewed and treated; they aren't only working to get a paycheck. If peer specialists don't view their role as an innovative disruptor educating mental health providers and peers then this isn't the job for them. Peers must get the support they need because they are working in a very complicated system. Peer specialists should be connected to the movement, either individually or collectively. They should understand the history and struggles of the movement and how it paved the way to where they are today.

The system will never be ready for this kind of thing

The perspective of Peter Stastny, the first psychiatrist to help implement peer-to-peer initiatives within mental health systems

For me, the Peer Specialist Project was inspired by a man who was a patient on the ward and then became the leader of a peer-operated food bank and outreach programme (Share Your Bounty). This man, William Brown, said: 'I used to be in the street preaching to people who have nothing. I was homeless, going crazy, and ended up in the hospital. But now I can turn things around and give back, and I can help these homeless people like I was helped.' We began to realise that people suddenly did better because they had a role, they had something meaningful to do, and they loved it. There was a woman on the ward who had been there for

20 years, and when they said, 'Do you want to make sandwiches for homeless people?' her whole demeanor changed. That's when I started to realise that stepping into a helper role really made a difference for people.

When you ask me if the project made a difference to the way things were done in and around the hospital, the short answer is no, it didn't affect it at all. Honestly, I saw some people working there as peer specialists who were worse than some of the staff; they wanted to be big shots and pull rank. That was not cool. They did it to impress the other workers.

The idea of peers working on an Assertive Community Treatment team (ACT) I would say now is a bad idea. They need to be really strong people in order to stand up to the system, and they've got to have the opportunity to change the way the team works. But in the current system, that's not possible.

At the time, there were also influences from the survivor movement, from Howie the Harp for example. He was the director of a peer-run drop-in centre for homeless people in Berkeley, California (Van Tosh & del Vecchio, 2000). Howie understood the needs of poor and homeless people, people who were on Skid Row, and at the same time he was very sophisticated in dealing with governments. He brought it all together. He was the one who said, 'We're really going to set up something to help those people that are down and out,' and that was where he came from. He was a labour organiser and a leftist, in the tradition of the Hobo movement of the 1930s.

But if you ask me whether peer specialists can change the system, I would say it's easier in places that are less controlled by institutional psychiatry. New York City is one of the places where institutional psychiatry has the most power. Maybe in other, less entrenched places, there might be more room. But then you might ask, 'What is it that would actually transform the system?' We're talking about a huge system, huge numbers of people who go into emergency rooms, hospitals, and all this. To make the experience different for a large number of them, you'd have to really turn things around. You'd have to create alternatives on a huge scale. They talk about scaling up this, scaling up that, but they're not talking about scaling up alternatives.

Back then we came up with some fairly radical stuff, but were stopped pretty soon. The only thing that survived was the Peer Specialist title. Everything else went by the wayside. We were the first to have a peer-run housing programme in New York State. We were the first to develop a peer-run technical assistance programme for people who want to start their own businesses and become economically self-sufficient. We had the first peer-run outreach programme for homeless people based at a mental institution. Those things all disappeared. One could say that we were ahead of our time, but one could also say that the system will never be ready for that kind of thing because it would mean giving up too much power.

What we learned from the project was that peer workers, ex-patients, have a tremendous ability to contribute. In the course of the project, and also through being introduced to the broader survivor movement, I saw the immense power of what people had to contribute. Another thing is that human beings are different. Just because you're an ICM worker doesn't mean you're automatically a bad person and just because you're a peer worker doesn't automatically mean you're a good person. I could tell you examples of people who worked as peer workers who were horrible, who were abusive, who were misogynistic. They're human beings, and people have talents and skills and flaws in addition to the experience and the knowledge that they have.

If I had to do it all over, I would put peer workers into situations where they could make more of a difference to a large number of people. If you give me a geographic region and say, 'Change the system,' I would say, 'Stand in the way of people getting admitted to the hospital. Stand in the doorway and provide something that's better for people, just as safe, but more helpful.'

I would like peers to be more involved in alternatives, and less involved in the system itself. I think that the system should heal itself, and I don't think that peers can do that for the system. There is too much of a burden on peers and the system is being let off the hook, because we're saying, 'OK, you hire some peers, and it'll be good to go.' That's nonsense. I see large hospital systems that hire a bunch of peers. They continue to do business as usual. Maybe people will have a better ride. It's possible. Obviously when you go to a jail, it's good to have conscientious people working there, instead of abusers, instead of people that will exploit you. If people have to go to a mental hospital they should be treated well. But it doesn't take peers to do that. It takes, again, human beings. So for the peers to be the conscience of the system, and for them to teach mental health professionals how to be decent human beings, and to listen, that's an undue burden.

Looking to the future

Peer specialists became role models based on their experiences as ex-patients and working with the ICM clients. Some of the clients wanted to become peer specialists just like us or move to other employment. This feeling of empowerment had a ripple effect with clients, the inpatients and outpatients at Bronx Psychiatric Center. The Peer Specialist Project led to real system change. The first peer specialist civil service title in New York State was approved. This led to many more peers being employed in the state mental health system. Other, non-profit programmes followed our lead and created similar peer specialist positions.

Setting a personal example was and still is one of the main attributes that peer specialists bring to the table, but that in and of itself it does not have systemic transformative power. Our peer specialists had no training in the behavioural sciences; they didn't know much about system theory or organisational development. In that sense, the expectation that peer workers alone would be a significant catalyst for change was far from reasonable.

Beyond the elusive goal of radical transformation, which may be a contradiction in terms when it comes to psychiatric institutions, involving and partnering with peers and peer-run organisations offers several benefits to peer providers as well as to the participants in such services. Needless to say, many ex-patients who have been sidelined from employment find welcome opportunities in working as service providers, and often respond quite favourably to these new roles where they are no longer at the receiving end of benefits. In the US, such positions have probably been the single most expanding opportunity in the job market for former psychiatric patients. This of course goes along with an improved social status, from beneficiary to provider of services, allowing many people to forgo their disability pensions and become eligible for mainstream social insurance programmes.

From the perspective of service participants – those who engage with peer-run or peer-provided services – many benefits have been reported anecdotally, and a smaller number have been borne out by more or less well-designed studies (Lloyd-Evans et al, 2012). Better service engagement, fewer involuntary hospitalisations, greater satisfaction with services, improved community integration, and a host of psychological variables such as empowerment, recovery orientation, a more hopeful, optimistic outlook for the future, fewer perceived problems, and enhanced quality of life in several areas have all been shown to result from engagement with peer support services.

The question of whether peer providers or peer-run organisations can actually reduce unwanted and traumatic experiences in mental health services is still unresolved. There are several studies of peer-run crisis centres that seem to support such a notion, but only one randomised controlled trial in California (Greenfield et al, 2008) has actually shown such positive effects. Nevertheless, satisfaction with peer-run crisis services is consistently greater than traditional ones, allowing us to extrapolate that there is overall less adversity and traumatisation in such services.

Clearly, involving peers in traditional services, whether they are meant to be working as 'change agents' or not, comes with a host of unwanted negative effects, such as co-optation by and collaboration with the system. This highly prevalent and nefarious development, which we have frequently witnessed, tends to occur either because the assigned role is structured to enhance the client/consumer's engagement with services they don't want (ie. ACT teams), or the hired peer is required to perform tasks that go against his/her value system. Either way, it is probably the single most important reason to be wary of such involvements. There are countless instances where peers have been brought into fundamentally problematic services, such as emergency rooms, ACT teams, even forensic services, where they frequently are positioned to 'soften the blow' or to put a better face on generally unpalatable measures. While the ethics of such involvement are highly problematic, ombudspeople (such as the service provided by peers in Sweden (Jesperson, 2007 and see Maths Jesperson's chapter in this book), and other forms of advocacy can also have an important protective role in precisely those situations.

One way to help distinguish co-opted from autonomous services is to identify the source of funding and the supervisory relationships. As long as there is a clear separation of fiscal and administrative authorities, co-optation may be kept at a minimum.

The draining of resources from the critical anti-psychiatry movement by engaging talented peers in the traditional system is highly troubling. Of course this is tied to the almost complete lack of funds for peer advocacy outside of mainstream mental health budgets. Therefore autonomous user-run organisations may be the best alternative to the absorption of all willing and talented ex-patients into the existing system and hoping they will exert transformative power.

But here too a lamentable development can be observed when large user-run outfits appear to specialise in certain functions that the mental health system doesn't mind shedding, such as social services, housing, legal advice, work training, where peers can make a difference, while traditional 'clinical' services are firmly kept in the hands of mental health professionals. This creates a two-tiered system, with the user-run organisations serving as lesser providers than their better trained (and better paid) colleagues.

There are a number of areas that need to be addressed if we are to move beyond the current state of affairs and see the development of truly successful and helpful collaborations. One is the integration of clinical and non-clinical services, with a strong, if not preponderant representation of peer voices. There are indeed examples of peer-run organisations where consumers/survivors can access a full range of psychosocial and peer support services, which may or may not be truly distinctive from those provided in traditional services. However, much further thought needs to be given to how such services can be truly distinct from traditional mental health services, protective of user rights, and responsive to the needs of persons seeking support.

References

Davidson L, Bellamy C, Guy K, Miller R (2012). Peer support among persons with severe mental illnesses: a review of evidence and experience. *World Psychiatry 11*(2): 123–128.

Felton CJ, Stastny P, Shern DL, Blanch A, Donahue SA, Knight E, Brown C (1995). Consumers as peer specialists on intensive case management teams: impact on client outcomes. *Psychiatric Services 46*(10): 1037–1044.

Greenfield TK, Stoneking BC, Humphreys K, Sundby E, Bond J (2008). A randomized trial of a mental health consumer-managed alternative to civil commitment for acute psychiatric crisis. *American Journal of Community Psychology 42*(1-2): 135–144.

Jesperson M (2007). Personal ombudsman in Skåne: a user-controlled service with personal agents. In: Stastny P, Lehmann P (eds). *Alternatives Beyond Psychiatry*. Berlin/Eugene, OR/Shrewsbury, UK: Peter Lehmann Publishing (pp161–167).

Lloyd-Evans B, Mayo-Wilson E, Harrison B, Istead H, Brown E, Pilling S, Johnson S, Kendall T (2014). A systematic review and meta-analysis of randomised controlled trials of peer support for people with severe mental illness. *BMC Psychiatry 14*: 39. Available at http://www.biomedcentral.com/1471-244X/14/39 (accessed 5 November, 2015).

Repper J, Carter T (2011). A review of the literature on peer support in mental health services. *Journal of Mental Health 20*(4): 392–411.

Stastny P, Brown C (2013). Pares especializados: orígenes, resultados, dificultades y diseminación a nivel mundial [Peer specialists: origins, outcomes, pitfalls and worldwide dissemination]. *Vertex 24*(112): 455–459.

Van Tosh L, del Vecchio P (2000). *Consumer/Survivor-Operated Self-Help Programs: a technical report. A retrospective review of the mental health consumer/survivor movement and 13 federally funded consumer/survivor-operated service programs in the 1980s*. Rockville, MD: US Department of Health and Human Services. Available at http://www.akmhcweb.org/docs/selfhelp.pdf (accessed 5 November, 2015).

21

Dilemmas of identity and power

Alison Faulkner

In this chapter I will draw on my experience in the research field and as a user/ survivor of mental health services to identify some of the dilemmas thrown up by working in partnership. The partnership I have in mind here is between service user or survivor researchers and academic or professional researchers who are not (usually) service users. We do not always fall neatly into these two distinct categories but for the purposes of this chapter I am interested in exploring what happens when these two groups of people come together to carry out research. For me these dilemmas are primarily about identity and power. Questions that confront us may be, for example: what identity am I assuming today or in the context of this piece of work? How do others see me? What influence do I or we have over this project? And what right do I have to do this research or to speak on behalf of others who are the subjects or participants of research?

In this chapter, I reflect on my experiences of six different research projects and on the issues they raise about identity and power.

Involvement, collaboration and control

Involvement in research is often conceptualised as a continuum from a more superficial consultation with service users (eg. asking people's views about a topic before constructing a questionnaire) through collaborative research to service user-controlled research. That intermediate level of 'collaboration' also has a continuum of its own and needs a bit of unpacking. A project may be truly collaborative, involving a partnership between service users and academic researchers, but in my experience that is quite rare. The collaboration I am more familiar with tends to start with the academic researchers reaching out to involve service users or survivor researchers in an already established project. This is not necessarily a problem, but it is vital to our shared understanding of where the decision-making power is located within the project, particularly when it comes to encountering difficulties and disagreements. The very language of 'involvement' implies that someone is or becomes involved in something else – there is a direction of movement implied in the word that is not implied, for example, by the term 'co-production'. Involvement does not sound like an equal partnership.

Figure 1:
A continuum of involvement

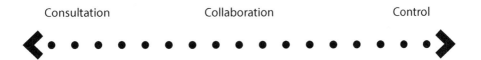

In thinking about these issues, I am drawing on my experience of six research projects (Table 1). In three of these projects (1, 4 and 6), I was directly involved as a researcher and/or trainer facilitating the involvement of other service users with less experience of research. In the remaining three projects (2, 3 and 5), I was involved in drawing together the learning from other people's research in different ways. In Beyond Our Expectations (project 2), I met and interviewed the researchers and service users involved in six projects in which users of forensic services were involved in research. In Changing Our Worlds (project 5), I interviewed the researchers and service users involved in seven user-controlled research projects that spanned a number of different health and disability themes. In the Colliding Worlds project (3), I facilitated an event that acted as closure for the researchers and service users involved after a particularly difficult experience of collaborative research.

(See next page for Table 1)

Table 1:
The research projects

1.	**Learning the Lessons:** an evaluation of community based services for people with a diagnosis of 'personality disorder' (Crawford et al, 2007).
2.	**Beyond our Expectations:** a report of the experiences of involving service users in forensic mental health research (Faulkner, 2006). The research was commissioned by a funding programme that is no longer in existence: the National Programme for Forensic Mental Health R&D.
3.	**A Story of Colliding Worlds:** a report capturing the experiences of the TRUE project (Faulkner, 2004). The report was commissioned by INVOLVE.
4.	**Getting Back into the World and Recovery Insights:** two reports of research (Ajayi et al, 2009; Bowyer et al, 2010) involving a team of service user researchers looking at service users' experiences of recovery. Both were commissioned by Rethink Mental Illness.
5.	**Changing Our Worlds:** examples of user-controlled research in action (Faulkner, 2010). The research was commissioned by INVOLVE.
6.	**Strategies for Living:** a report of user-led research into people's strategies for living with mental distress (Faulkner & Layzell, 2000). The report was one product to emerge from a six-year programme (1997–2003) of user-led research and capacity building for service users wishing to do their own research. The final report was published by the Mental Health Foundation and is now out of print.

The six pieces of work lie at different places along that imaginary continuum of involvement. At the 'user-controlled' end are Strategies for Living and Changing Our Worlds, projects in which service users (or disabled people) as researchers had significant, if not complete, control over the research being carried out. These examples contain some inspiring instances of empowerment and achievement, along with some significant struggles, such as encountering stigma/discrimination and a desperate lack of resources.

In the centre of the continuum are the recovery research of Rethink Mental Illness and the collection of case studies in Beyond Our Expectations. However, this is where the continuum begins to break down. A couple of the projects featured in Beyond Our Expectations could be classified as user-led, but all of them struggled for power and control within forensic mental health settings, where even academic researchers can encounter barriers. The Rethink Mental Illness recovery research was a good example of collaborative research, and perhaps the best I have come across in my personal experience. The service user researchers worked with the non-service user research project manager, each contributing from their own expertise and taking a full part in the data collection, analysis and interpretation. However this research challenges our ethical principles in other ways because it was funded by a pharmaceutical company and, although the research was not influenced by the company on a day-to-day level, the knowledge that we were funded by a drug company lurked in the background.

Moving towards the consultation end of the continuum are Learning the Lessons and the Colliding Worlds project. Again, the simplistic nature of the continuum fails us. In the former, I had the privilege of being involved in one module of this large programme of work, the module being led by a service user research team based at the Mental Health Foundation. It was a rigorous piece of work carried out with integrity and a significant degree of service user control. However it was only one module out of four; the rest (and the programme as a whole) were led by academic researchers and so our single module did not have as much status or impact as it might have done. In Colliding Worlds I listened to, and learned from, researchers and service users about some of the issues that arise when a collaboration does not work well – issues of power and identity writ large. A group of service users had been involved in research to look at the training available nationally for patients, carers and service users to get involved in research, but their own team had suffered from profound divisions and difficulties.

Reflections

Reflecting on the findings and experiences from these diverse pieces of work, I identified the following themes as features that might help us to move from involvement to partnership – or, to borrow from Colliding Worlds, to move from colliding to collaborative worlds:

- understanding power and inequalities
- attitudes – eg. respect, acceptance
- clear roles and expectations
- adequate time and resources
- accessibility – eg. language, payments (readily available cash reimbursements)
- support and supervision throughout
- being involved from the start
- constructive means of negotiation.

If we can put these ingredients into the collaboration 'pot', then I believe that we can achieve great things out of working in partnership. For example:

- new knowledge and theory
- sharing the research gaze
- empowerment
- confidence and skills
- trust between the researcher and the researched – leading to better quality research
- asking the right questions – based on the insight and knowledge gained from personal experience – leading to better quality information
- making change happen – based on the increased quality of research but also on the commitment of service users to enabling change to happen
- highlighting the issues of importance to diverse and marginalised communities
- using our own experiences to shed light on the results, analysis and interpretation of the results.

I was struck by the language of the titles of the reports – that three of them refer in some way to our 'world' or 'worlds'. This led me to think about the different world-views that can be represented in involvement activities. Engagement in 'user involvement', whether in research or other activities, is both a personal and a political enterprise: political in that we do want to change some aspect of the mental health world, and personal in that we bring sometimes painful and humiliating aspects of our personal lives and experiences to bear on the activity we are involved in.

This does not always fit well with the project or enterprise concerned, whether it be research or service development. Those whose job it is to plan and run services or to conduct research may not be familiar with the entirety of experience that service users often bring with them into an involvement activity. They may be relating to others from within their work or professional roles, whereas we may be bringing our life experiences, our identities, to bear on the activity. I think this can lead to a profound mismatch in motivation and understandings. It can make the effort of working in partnership, or working collaboratively, at the very least problematic. We can find ourselves feeling, and being accused of being, emotional in unfamiliar work environments where those around us are operating in administrative or bureaucratic ways. This was particularly evident in the Colliding Worlds project, but is not an unfamiliar experience.

> *You're bringing together worlds which up to now have collided... so you have the academic world versus the patient or service user world – where we've had everything done to us over the last few years and decades... So it's this idea that you've got all these different worlds colliding and none of us have the answers for how to facilitate that (service user quoted in Faulkner, 2004).*

Identity and power?

It is not just about identity and power. The different partners can enter into an involvement activity with very different, sometimes contradictory, motivations. Clinical academics in a research project are likely to be as much motivated by career ambition and the need to achieve the markers of research success, such as publications and future funding bids, as they are by the desire to 'do good' with their research. Service users are usually motivated by the desire to change and improve things for their extended communities, to 'change their worlds' or some part of the mental health world for themselves and for future service users. This is a somewhat simplistic characterisation, as we all have mixed motives in these situations, but it often holds true.

Diana Rose has described service user involvement in research (her own and that of others) as people embodying madness and irrationality engaged in what is essentially a rational enterprise, and suggests that for some clinical academic researchers this is just too much of a challenge (Rose, 2003):

> *Among the many ways that power manifests itself in medical research is when senior academics do not treat a service user as a research collaborator, and simply regard the person as somebody's (a potential?) patient. I have been in research meetings that suddenly felt like a ward round. One's user status may be used to undermine one's opinions, as it is held that a person cannot be both logical and mad. It is a difficult balance to strike – that having a diagnosis and experience of services is a qualification for the job and not a handicap. This is the reverse side of the value of a double identity, and I do not pretend to have resolved the issue.*

I have had this experience myself – I walked into a seminar where I was due to speak on acute mental health care to find a psychiatrist in the audience who had once admitted me to hospital. I wanted the ground to open up beneath my feet. But, having got over that initial reaction, I managed to speak to her later and she was entirely supportive of my being there and talking about what it is like to be in hospital. It seemed that she, too, was deeply unhappy with the nature of acute mental health care.

However, as Diana also concedes, the wearing of two hats (researcher and service user) can sometimes mean that we can be less accepted within the service user world too. People can struggle to believe in your 'service user' status or may see you as something of a traitor who has crossed over into the academic world and is siding with those who see service users as patients and research fodder, rather than as individuals and potential research partners.

This has, I believe, a number of implications for what can happen. We have seen that in some cases it leads to 'colliding worlds', with differences, dissent and distress becoming the dominant experience for everybody. However it can lead to a shared and more holistic understanding of those worlds if both parties can work together. But it means that an awareness of these different world-views/perspectives and the inherent power differentials is vital. A willingness to listen, to learn and to change and to compromise – from everyone – is essential to the success of partnership working.

Like many other survivor researchers, I do not have any easy answers for how this is best worked out in practice. I only know that we all need to be aware of where the power lies. In the work that I carried out for Changing our Worlds, in which I met several service users and disabled people who had carried out user-controlled research, I became newly aware of the importance of power. These seven projects were all small scale studies that had achieved a great deal of impact with remarkably little in the way of resources. They had sought to raise awareness of the issues affecting groups and communities of people whose voices are rarely heard, and they had nearly all achieved this. They had each shone a light into a small, dark corner previously unexplored by mainstream research.

In the process of doing this, one of the researchers, a deaf woman, had come to understand the complexities of her new role and status. As both researcher and service user, she had come to assume a position of power in relation to the service users she interviewed for the research, and yet, paradoxically, she had no power to effect change in their immediate situation. This affected her deeply:

I want to get my research skills up, report writing and things, but I am aware that I'm growing in power. I've only realised it recently because of getting into emancipatory research. It's like I'm being paid, but you [the interviewee] are the one who is still having to go through it (quoted in Faulkner, 2010: 50).

Another disabled researcher, engaged in examining people's experiences of disability hate crime, became the victim of hate crime himself during the course of the research, having been shouted at and abused as he left one of the research interviews.

Those of us who wear (at least) two hats – researcher and service user/ survivor – have a particular responsibility. We have to both uphold the value of service users as equal partners in the research process and uphold the value of good quality research. We can perhaps become a bridge between those worlds. However, in the effort to straddle these worlds, we have to try not to fall through the gaps between them; instead, we need to find ways of bringing them together and forging greater understandings.

One of the issues that might cause us to fall through the gaps is our tendency to neglect research and researchers from black and minority ethnic (BME) communities. When searching for examples of user-controlled research for the Changing Our Worlds project, we did not find any examples from BME health or disability researchers. As white service user/survivor researchers, then, we have the responsibility to acknowledge that we are telling only part of the story. We have a responsibility not to replicate the mistakes made by mainstream mental health research by neglecting the issues that affect BME service users and survivors. Identity and power are issues of particular significance to black and other marginalised and minority communities.

Collaborative research, or involvement in research, comes in many different forms, as these examples illustrate. The continuum in Figure 1 cannot do justice to the variety of different ways in which service users or survivors come to take part in research. There continue to be barriers that prevent us from realising our potential to contribute to the production of mental health knowledge and meaningful evidence. All too often, the involvement of service users in other people's research is tokenistic and is sanitised to the point that it is rendered meaningless (Russo, 2012). But there are examples of good and productive collaborative research, where partnerships are meaningful and respectfully examined (eg. Gillard et al, 2012). Unfortunately the systems that exist do not allow us to distinguish easily between these before we become involved; it is still rare for service users to become involved in research before the proposal has been submitted, so relationships cannot be formed in advance and decisions made accordingly. We have little choice but to accept this if we really want to take part and we do not have the power to change things after the proposal has been accepted. We need to build our own networks of knowledge and information and support others who become involved in research, both to share the experience of good partnerships and to shout more loudly when things go wrong. Better than that, we need more resources to carry out our own survivor research.

References

Ajayi S, Bowyer T, Hicks A, Larsen J, Mailey P, Sayers R, Smith R, two anonymous authors (2009). *Getting Back into the World: reflections on lived experiences of recovery*. Rethink recovery series volume 2. London: Rethink.

Bowyer T, Hicks A, Mailey P, Sayers R, Smith R, Ajayi S, Faulkner A, Larsen J, two anonymous authors. *Recovery Insights: learning from experience*. Rethink recovery series volume 3. London: Rethink; 2010.

Crawford M, Rutter D, Price K, Weaver T, Josson M, Tyrer P et al (2007). *Learning the Lessons: a multi-method evaluation of dedicated community-based services for people with personality disorder*. Report for the National Co-ordinating Centre for NHS Service Delivery and Organisation R&D (NCCSDO). London: HMSO; 2007.

Crawford MJ, Rutter D, Manley C, Bhui K, Weaver T, Fulop N, Tyrer P (2001). *User Involvement in the Planning and Delivery of Mental Health Services: a report to London Region NHSE*. London: National Health Service Executive.

Faulkner A (2010). *Changing our Worlds: examples of user-controlled research in action*. Eastleigh: INVOLVE. Available at www.invo.org.uk (accessed 28 October, 2015).

Faulkner A (2006). *Beyond our Expectations: a report of the experiences of involving service users in forensic mental health research*. London: National Programme for Forensic Mental Health R&D, Department of Health. Available at www.invo.org.uk (accessed 28 October, 2015).

Faulkner A (2004). *Capturing the Experiences of the TRUE Project: a story of colliding worlds*. Eastleigh: INVOLVE. Available at www.invo.org.uk (accessed 28 October, 2015).

Faulkner A, Layzell S (2000). *Strategies for Living: a report of user-led research into people's strategies for living with mental distress*. London: Mental Health Foundation. Summary available at www.mentalhealth.org.uk/content/assets/PDF/publications/strategies_for_living_summary.pdf (accessed 28 October, 2015).

Faulkner A, Gillespie S, Imlack S, Dhillon K, Crawford M (2008). Learning the lessons together. *Mental Health Today* 8(1): 24–26.

Gillard S, Simons L, Turner K, Lucock M, Edwards C (2012). Patient and public involvement in the coproduction of knowledge: reflection on the analysis of qualitative data in a mental health study. *Qualitative Health Research* 22(8): 1126–1137.

Lindow V (2001). Survivor research. In: Newnes C, Holmes G, Dunn C (eds). *This is Madness Too*. Ross-on-Wye: PCCS Books (pp135–146).

Rose D (2003). Having a diagnosis is a qualification for the job. *British Medical Journal* 326(7402): 1331.

Russo J (2012). Survivor-controlled research: a new foundation for thinking about psychiatry and mental health. *Forum: Qualitative Social Research* 13(1): Art. 8. http://nbn-resolving.de/urn:nbn:de:0114-fqs120187 (accessed 28 October, 2015).

22

Is partnership a dirty word?

Cath Roper

In this chapter I use my experiences as a consumer academic employed at the University of Melbourne's Centre for Psychiatric Nursing as a case study through which to examine critically the nature of partnerships and their potential within academia. Both the Centre for Psychiatric Nursing and the consumer academic role are funded by the Department of Health, Victoria, Australia. The simple angle I am taking on this topic is that partnerships in psychiatry are political. This chapter raises questions about whether 'equal' work relationships with non-consumers are possible or whether they are even a desirable goal. I argue that our work partnerships in psychiatry depend on identifying and attending to inequality and positioning us as unique and necessary thinkers, knowers and leaders in the development of quality work. Our allies therefore have a role in facilitating material conditions and environments conducive to the growth of our leadership and the growth of consumer knowledge.

The chapter begins by briefly addressing the establishment of the consumer academic role, then analyses structural and individual issues pertaining to the conduct of the role. Finally affirmative action techniques are explored that make our partnerships more likely to work.

Emergence of the consumer academic role

The world's-first (to my knowledge) designated consumer-perspective academic post was established in 2000. It was the product of a partnership between the Centre for Psychiatric Nursing and the Melbourne Consumer Consultants Group, an incorporated, independent group of consumer consultants. Together they sought funding for the innovative role from the Commonwealth Department of Health and Aged Care. Rather than placing significance on academic qualification, the position title *consumer academic* was intended to describe the *setting* where the consumer was working (academia), in the same way that the term *consumer consultant* described a consumer role within a mental health service setting.

The inaugural Director of the Centre for Psychiatric Nursing, Professor Brenda Happell, had been present at a national initiative known as 'the Deakin workshops' (Deakin Human Services Australia, 1999), which were held in 1998 in response to research findings that consumers found the attitudes of mental health professionals to be at least as debilitating for their recovery as any 'symptoms' they were experiencing. The Deakin workshops comprised equal numbers of individuals from all disciplines in mental health, including consumers and carers (Grey, 2014). Happell became convinced that the consumer perspective[1] could and should be embedded within the academic setting because '… consumers of mental health services needed genuine opportunities to influence the attitudes of mental health professionals through active involvement in the education process' (Happell & Roper, 2009: 575).

For many attendees it was a watershed experience that would spawn lasting partnerships and give impetus to new ways for consumers to influence the professional development of clinicians. Happell went on to establish other roles for consumer educators and academics across Australia and is a leading advocate for consumer perspective and consumer leadership in academia.

Partnerships are political

Structural issues

Whether consciously perceived at the time or not, the consumer academic role was a political strategy to tackle discriminatory attitudes held by clinicians. But the reality was that a lone, half-time consumer position, charged with

---

1. The term 'consumer perspective' used in this chapter is based on Epstein and Shaw's (1997) definition. While they acknowledge the difficulty of pinning down 'consumer perspective', they imbue it with ideas about belonging to a socio-political movement, having solidarity and a shared identity through collective experience of marginalisation, discrimination and oppression. The phrase suggests a particular lens through which experience is viewed. In addition, 'consumer perspective' is the term used here to describe an emerging academic discipline.

influencing clinicians' attitudes and located within a clinical academic setting, would inevitably be a tough gig – for two related reasons: the personal safety of the consumer academic, and the level of influence possible in the role. A project team with a consumer majority was established as an initial strategy to support the role and 'keep it real', so the post holder did not become seduced by 'life in the ivory tower' of academia. With hindsight, however, there was a fundamental flaw in the way the role was set up: its implicit function as an advocacy tool for the consumer movement at times placed it in conflict with ideas about 'rigour' and 'impartiality' in the academic setting.

The Centre for Psychiatric Nursing is situated in a positivist scientific, evidence-based paradigm. Its overall programme of work is centred on physical health and medication safety in the context of mental health nursing in Victorian public mental health service settings. It favours quantitative research approaches and reproduces the 'dominant medicalised individual discourse' (Russo & Beresford, 2014: 1) through its research programmes and professional development activity. In contrast, I have a background in teaching rather than research or the healthcare professions. I identify as a *survivor* of mental health services (even if this is not always the word I use) and it is publicly known that my mental health services use has been involuntary.

One example where, despite the best intentions, messages can be lost in translation is the furore among some mental health clinicians over the 'Batty is beautiful' t-shirts that I designed as a fundraiser, which depicted a rather cheeky bat looking out from behind his/her folded wings. For some clinicians, Batty represented the worst example of discriminatory attitudes. To me, and to the wearers of Batty t-shirts, it was a mark of pride, not shame.

The relationship between the setting and the incumbent in the consumer academic role and its impact on broader work relations might be idiosyncratic. However, broader structural analyses can be made. For example, levels of influence and safety are inherently problematic with part-time work. It is problematic if there is a head-on collision between subjective and objective knowledge in a setting where less value is placed on subjective knowledge or if a lay perspective is ostensibly sought but not respected in the hierarchy of professional knowledges. Trying to exert influence as the sole 'representative' in any situation risks marginalisation. Lack of influence itself can become internalised as a personal fault rather than analysed as a structural problem, and this can further compound personal unsafety. More specifically, consumers often bring the knowledge and expertise they have acquired from their experiences to inform their work – experiences that are often underlaid by a significant trauma background. Many consumers have also experienced 'sanctuary harm' (Robins et al, 2005; Grubaugh et al, 2007) – that is, trauma that has been induced by iatrogenic service use. As a consequence of my own experiences, for instance, I can never take for granted sovereignty over my body or trust that my wishes will be respected. It means that in work situations my body is like a barometer, constantly on the alert for unsafety; my body tells me, for example, when something is ethically wrong, through physical sensations.

Miranda Fricker's (2007) concept of 'epistemic injustice' is also relevant to the issue of personal safety. Epistemic injustice occurs when a 'knower' is 'wronged in their capacity to know' – when a listener fails to give a proper hearing (discounts the person) through prejudice. As an example, epistemic injustice occurs when the testimony of a person with a psychiatric diagnosis is doubted on grounds that they must be irrational, fantasising, lying, not able to discern truth etc. Fricker says: 'Where it goes deep, it can cramp self-development, so that a person may be, quite literally, prevented from becoming who they are' (2007: 5). When all of these factors are put together, it is not surprising that there are significant issues of personal safety in the consumer academic role and these in turn affect the work relationships established in the role. Such issues may be only partially visible or be entirely invisible and it may be hard to hold onto structural analyses. All of this can in turn impact on the experience of having influence in the consumer academic role.

Strategies

One answer to some of the structural issues identified above is to ensure some aspects of the work are controlled by the consumer academic. Another strategy is to ensure that some of the work is 'consumer-only'. The consumer academic role would not exist and nothing could be achieved in it without the support of non-consumer allies and consumers, both individually and collectively. When we do partner, it is with allies who have demonstrated their commitment to consumer leadership and consumer perspectives. One such example (both consumer controlled and transdisciplinary) is the Psych Action and Training (PAT) group. The Centre for Psychiatric Nursing provides material support for the development of consumer leadership and consumer perspective in academia through funding consumer members to attend the group. PAT provides its members with a supportive space to discuss our work and work environments through a critical lens, resulting in the potential for helpful structural analyses and the development of new knowledge.

The fact that my experience of mental health services has been involuntary influences the scope and content of all my work, the partnerships that are open to me, the allies I seek out, and the work opportunities with which I will and won't get involved. For example, involvement in research into practices to reduce and eliminate seclusion and restraint and co-leading research into offering consumers a post-seclusion or restraint 'testimonial space' is in tune with my experience, interests and expertise. Similarly, two projects on which I am working with colleagues at the Centre for Psychiatric Nursing are developing supported decision-making training (Roper, Hopkins & Houghton, 2014) and sharing the project management of the Tools for Change Recovery Library.[1] These developments have only been made possible through mutual commitment to having the kinds of honest and at times uncomfortable conversations alluded to in the sections that follow.

Is partnership possible or desirable?

It could be argued that the concept of 'partnership' is a flawed way to describe work relations between consumers and non-consumers because of its focus on mutual co-operation and responsibility. This notion of mutuality in the context of unequal power is likely to contribute to disguising inequalities that are present. More crucially, it does not acknowledge the heroic lengths to which consumers may have to go to stay present in work if they have experienced forced treatment yet are working alongside service providers who represent the source of that trauma and oppression.

Another way to look at partnerships in psychiatry is to start by acknowledging that they are not equal and to shift the focus away from equality to a commitment to articulating inequality. It requires acceptance that a level playing field, with consumers being just one of many (equal) players, is a fantasy, as is the idea that all consumers are a homogenous group. There will be a variety of relative social, institutional or other advantages and privileges that will need to be identified, acknowledged and ameliorated. If this work does not happen, there is a danger that those with less power will bear the burden of whatever is unspoken. Establishing spaces where consumers can share their structural analyses with each other can help name and offset inequalities.

Affirmative action techniques

Placing consumer knowledge at the heart of partnerships

If we assume partnerships are not equal, new questions emerge. What can be learned about relative inequality and how do we deal with it throughout this

---

1. See www.recoverylibrary.unimelb.edu.au

partnership? What if some partners are using knowledge derived from trauma experiences in the work they do? What does it mean for the partnership if some of the partners have multiple experiences of powerlessness and lack of voice and yet this is simultaneously the motivation for their involvement? What structures might need to be put in place so that these experiences can be explored openly, converted into mutual learning and given primacy? What if some of the partners have such finely tuned radars for injustice that they undergo somatic responses, blanking out, freezing or feeling sick? How will that be noted and a space created where words can be found and experiences articulated? If these kinds of issues have been discussed by all partners from the outset (on the basis that these reactions are precious and informative, not personally weak and shameful), there is more chance they will be recognised as signs that something in the work or in the partnership itself has gone off the rails, and it is not an individual malady. There is great potential for new knowledge to be created from re-orienting how we think about partnerships and asking these kinds of questions.

Paying close attention to the reactions of the least powerful people 'in the room' may take more time but it is an essential element of working together and something all partners can learn and benefit from. As an example, consumers often have an awareness that emotions are an inevitable part of work, whereas expectations of being 'professional' tend to emphasise being dispassionate. Knowledge we might have about strong feelings and emotional sensitivity and about techniques we have learned that give them proper place generally goes untapped, yet it could so easily be capitalised on as an asset in partnership work. To work this way is not 'therapy' (Epstein & Olsen, 1998: 44); it is political and it is about producing quality work that crucially decreases the chances of consumers (and indeed everyone) being harmed.

Consumers not only have unique and necessary knowledge to offer; we often have well-developed, healthy and ethical work processes that are of universal benefit. When our knowledge is placed at the heart of partnerships there is enormous potential for further theory development and articulation of consumer perspectives. The fundamental questions are: what do consumers bring to the partnership or to the work that nobody else can bring? What is the particular expertise they have that is needed/desired?

Practical questions

Explicit goals of working together can be the enrichment and promotion of consumer leadership and the broader development of consumer capacity. The following questions are about attending to power in partnerships with consumers and can be used as prompts for discussion in preparation for beginning work, and as reminders throughout the course of any initiative.

- Does this endeavour further the aims of the consumer movement, or of the consumers who are using this service, or of the consumers who have a strong interest in this work?
- Has the agenda been decided by consumers, or with them as part of the partnership, or has it been decided beforehand without the consumers?
- If consumers are not leading the partnership, is there investment in the development of consumer leadership?
- How much influence do the consumers have over the direction of the work and how would they know? Do they have power of veto? Is their voice heard and how would that be proved? If not, how will the situation be redressed so that tokenism, harm or re-inscription of powerlessness and voicelessness are avoided and to equalise the power and influence consumers have?
- What does each partner bring to the partnership and what can they learn from it?
- How do we make visible issues of voice, power, who has it and when?
- Does the partnership create opportunities for consumer capacity development (eg. training, mentorship, career development, creation of consumer groups, networks, employment or study opportunities)?

Practical strategies

Practical strategies for affirmative action include setting up processes whereby consumers can determine the priorities for work and set the agenda. Preparation is also important in partnerships with non-consumers. One practical preparation strategy is to seek the advice of consumers with partnership experience because they are likely to know how to audit work environments and can identify and advise on any participatory structures needed. They will have links with consumer organisations, can review supervision and debriefing structures and can help with setting up consumer-only spaces and so on. They can also advise on how to minimise the likelihood of unethical practice – how to ensure that consumers are not being set up or employed in tokenistic positions, for example, and that partnership processes are transparent and accountable.

The role of allies

Our allies are prepared to disturb the status quo. They work with us to promote consumer perspective and they help make space for it. They create agency for us, provide mentorship when we need it and create opportunities for us to lead. They use their influence, institutional power and networks to harness and grow consumer leadership. They facilitate the turning of administrative wheels, such as ensuring timely payment. They are on the lookout for funding opportunities for forthcoming work and dissemination opportunities for completed work. They understand powerful feelings are real and are not to be pitted against rationality – they understand that many of us have experienced 'epistemic injustice' and have had our analyses ignored. If they involve us in their work, it happens from the beginning. Our allies want to know our agenda. They know that consumer perspective is unique and has much to teach others. We trust our allies because we have had many difficult conversations with them and we will go on to have many more. These partnerships are many years in the making.

Conclusion

Like all marginalised groups, we are likely to be carrying deep experiences of oppressive structures and be susceptible to the ongoing legacy of those experiences. I see this not as a source of shameful weakness, however, but as the source of our greatest untapped strength, because it is possible for us to use the visceral knowledge we hold to create new types of environments that work well for everybody and that support the development of new approaches to partnership that are attentive and alive to power.

References

Deakin Human Services Australia (1999). *Learning Together: education and training partnerships in mental health*. Canberra, ACT: Commonwealth Department of Health and Aged Care. http://webarchive.nla.gov.au/gov/20110403053320/https://www.health.gov.au/internet/main/publishing.nsf/Content/mental-pubs-l-learn (accessed 31 January, 2015)

Epstein M, Olsen A (1998). An introduction to consumer politics. *Journal of Psychosocial and Mental Health Services* 36(8): 40–49.

Epstein M, Shaw J (1997). *Developing Effective Consumer Participation in Mental Health Services: the report of the Lemon Tree Learning Project*. Brunswick: Victorian Mental Illness Awareness Council.

Fricker M (2007). *Epistemic Injustice: power and the ethics of knowing.* Oxford: Oxford University Press.

Grey F (2014). *Consumers as Educators, Some Historical Context.* [Online.] Melbourne: Department of Nursing, Melbourne University. http://nursing.unimelb.edu.au/consumerinvolvementstation/context_history (accessed 21 December, 2014).

Grubaugh AL, Frueh BC, Zinzow HM, Cusack KJ, Wells C (2007). Patients' perceptions of care and safety within psychiatric settings. *Psychological Services 4*(3): 193–201.

Happell B, Roper C (2009). Promoting genuine consumer participation in mental health education: a consumer academic role. *Nurse Education Today 29*(6): 575–579.

Robins CS, Sauvageot JA, Cusack KJ, Suffoletta-Maierle S, Frueh BC (2005). Consumers' perceptions of negative experiences and 'sanctuary harm' in psychiatric settings. *Psychiatric Services 56*(9): 1134–1138.

Roper C, Hopkins F, Houghton J (2014). 'Who's got the wheel?' Consumer leadership and co-production in the training of mental health clinicians. [Online.] *Health Issues 113*(Summer): 34–37. http://search.informit.com.au/documentSummary;dn=834953258220146;res=IELHEA (accessed 12 November, 2015).

Russo J, Beresford P (2014). Between exclusion and colonisation: seeking a place for mad people's knowledge in academia. *Disability & Society 30*(1): 153–157.

23

Co-creating the ways we carry each other: reflections on being an ally and a double agent

Reima Ana Maglajlic

First things first – I am deeply honoured to contribute to this book on real alternatives to psychiatry. Particularly as I always think that a) I didn't do much, and b) that I should have done and should do much more. I was invited, I guess, with my 'ally' hat on and because of the work I did in Bosnia and Herzegovina in the late 1990s and better part of the 2000s, supporting the development of survivor-run initiatives in mental health and, for a little while, supporting the development of community-based mental health services in the same country. Before that I was in England, learning my craft as a social worker from one of the first mental-health-system-survivors-cum-professors-of-social-work, the late Professor David Brandon. This was not a random event – I wanted to learn from him and did just that for five years, having packed my bags and moved from Croatia to England.

I thought long and hard about the key things I should focus on, based not just on these experiences but on the past 20 years of my involvement in social work and social care. Summed up, it may come down to several things. First, I wouldn't mind sharing a word or two of musings on identity and labelling in relation to alternatives to psychiatry. Second, I wish to do the same in relation to why I think we have lost sight of the bigger picture, and why, by losing it, decades after the first alternatives were developed, we are still injecting, medicating and isolating far more than supporting each other or embracing madness as part of our fabric. Both are related to our values, whether these be professional or private, and what we intend to do with our time and leave behind us. Finally, I won't necessarily talk about it in that particular order. I shall start with a few snippets of experiences that may have led me to this book.

Alan's revolution

I am in the middle of a rave party in a field somewhere in England. I have lost Alan.[1] A few days before, his entire demeanour had changed. He joined a revolution that only he could see. All I knew was that he was in front of the barricades and I was lagging behind. This was an era before mobile phones, before professional registration, when care in the community was in full swing in the UK, haloperidol ruled, and risperidone was just becoming the new drug of choice to calm people like him. I never liked any of the meds and neither did Alan. But at that party, I wished I had a massive injection just to calm his pace. I hated myself for it. We lost him. He was detained and sectioned. It was either us or the police, whoever got to him first.

Alan wasn't an exception; it's a pretty standard mid-1990s story of how our society dealt with madness, and particularly (the real) mad men. Many experiences are, unfortunately, similar even today. What we were experimenting with wasn't that novel, but it seemed that way to us. Could we prevent Alan from going into hospital, keep him with us – his friends, or me, his girlfriend? Before he rejoined the revolution that only he experienced, we tried to start drafting a crisis plan. What he would like to happen. When 'the revolution started', we tried to stick with the plan. It didn't work that time. I have seen what it looks like when it does work. I know people who have been supported by community-based crisis teams comprising friends, family, volunteers, even professionals (as in people paid to offer some form of support). I am not going to cite a randomised controlled trial to prove it, but I know what such support looks like and that it can work.

Changes in Bosnia and Herzegovina

Cut to an advocacy training event for survivor organisations in Bosnia, an emerging network at that time. No, cut to several years earlier. In the late 1990s, a friend of mine, one of the founders of the survivor movement in Slovenia, told me that something good, something important, was happening in Bosnia and

---

1. This is a pseudonym.

Herzegovina (BiH). When it comes to such insights, I trust no one like I trust people who have survived mental health services. I lived in England at the time. And I wanted to go home, to south-east Europe.

BiH never had big mental health institutions, at least not as big as the ones in neighbouring Croatia and Serbia, with a thousand-plus people imprisoned in them. People in BiH who had the misfortune to be labelled 'chronically' mad and for whom there were no beds 'locally' (I use the word loosely, as the 'local' bed could actually be hundreds of kilometres away) would be shipped out of the country to one of the neighbouring, at the time federal, states. The most positive thing that happened during the 1991–1996 war was that the majority of the psychiatric hospitals that did exist got bombed – and without anyone in them at the time. It is one way to start a reform. And it did.

There were other, equally important factors. During the war, international organisations descended on the region like a plague. But some of them actually managed to do good. The WHO office in Bosnia was at the time run by Italian doctors who had worked on the reform of Italian mental health services. When they were offered funding to support the rebuilding of the psychiatric hospitals, they decided to spend it on the development of community mental health services instead. There were also two local eminent psychiatrists who had trained at the Maudsley Hospital in the UK, and who understood that this would be a good idea. There was a good team at one of the key Ministries of Health (BiH has 13 layers of governance, each with legislative and other decision-making powers), and one of the doctors had set up primary care mental health services. Any change, any alternative, needs allies. I packed my bags; I wanted to be part of that.

Finding allies and learning from a madness Jedi master

Two other significant things followed that helped with the creation of survivor-run initiatives. The UK-based organisation Hamlet Trust[2] was still in existence. This was a network of initiatives led or run by mental health system survivors across 18 countries in south-east and eastern Europe and the former Soviet Union, with more than 50 member organisations. Without their funding and support none of the survivor groups would have been developed or sustained. And I like knocking on doors. My first was the door to the day centre in Sarajevo University Hospital. There were a number of people who had got a taste of better

---

2. The organisation no longer exists, but some information is available at www.hamlettrust.plus.com/about.html

health care through being both mad and refugees in other countries. A couple of them wanted to start a local survivor-run group. We heard that there was a similar group in a day hospital in Tuzla, in north-east Bosnia. I paid for the three of us to go together for a visit. Tuzla was and is a special place. From that group at the day hospital, a 'Fenix' emerged in more ways than one – it is now the only remaining survivor-run group in BiH. Also, a few dedicated and supportive doctors worked at the Tuzla day hospital who wanted to do things differently and were battling against any attempt to open new hospitals and lobbying for funds to go to setting up community-based support services.

We all need allies, no matter what we do. Just a few months earlier I had tried to find them in Zagreb, Croatia – my home town. There was one psychiatrist who was trying to start a support group and was fighting for the recognition that psychiatrists are inherently bad seeds, based on the example of Radovan Karadzic (google him, I'd better not go there), but who was still referring to schizophrenics and manic-depressives. There was no one else.

Now I've started writing this down, many memories come back, but it's best I don't share them all. Some are good and some not so much. Some are funny; madness has that intense, surreal quality and you have to have a good laugh with it at least once in a while. Some hurt and were very scary for everyone involved.

Cut back to the advocacy training. It was mainly conducted by other mental health system survivors from other countries in south-east Europe and from the UK. One of them felt he might not be able to go through with it. He gave us strict instructions as to how to treat him and what he needed in terms of support. This included cancelling some of his commitments, but he also asked to be locked in a room overnight, to prevent him wandering off, and to be provided with enough pens and paper to last him through the night. We followed all his instructions to the letter. The man was an expert in his own madness and how to direct people around him. It was a thing of beauty and an exercise in self-control that I have only ever come across with other people in a similar situation who have had similar crisis support. Because of him and several similar experiences, I know that informal and community crisis support does work. But it takes time. This was his 'crisis' number four or five – not the first one. He was already a Jedi master of his own madness. There was another thing that mattered – he wanted to compromise. He loved his madness, but he also loved people around him who, just like me with Alan, couldn't keep up. He compromised to keep them near, because they were as important to him as he was to them. Alan didn't want to, no matter how hard we both tried.

Co-creating what we know

In parallel with supporting the development of survivor-run initiatives, I made sure that, when studies were conducted on the progress of the community mental health reform in BiH, people with experience of using these services were part of the study as stakeholders, not objects. They were involved in defining the methodology, conducting interviews, making sense of the data, the lot. They were also part of the teaching staff on the Community Mental Health MA for social workers, psychologists and psychiatrists (which was my day job throughout). I also tried to open a drop-in at our space at the University of Sarajevo (and we succeeded, for about a year, before they kicked us out). I ensured that BiH was included in the Tower Hamlets 'Pathways to Policy' project (Cutler & Hayward, 2005), which led to a number of employment initiatives, thanks to the devotion and hard work of the members of Fenix, the local survivor-run initiative, and, for a short period of time, to transition housing provision. None of it could have happened had I not had strong local allies. I just happened to open some doors.

I tried to support the development of a different way of being and doing, working either on my own or with others and putting them in touch with each other. In BiH, much gets easily lost in the quicksand of development funding, projectisation, eternal transition and through some of the pieces of the support puzzle going missing. It plagues me that so little of this survives. This is an ongoing, Sisyphus job. It takes allies and it takes time, a lot of it.

One episode of Star Trek too many

Why do I do it in the first place? I have given this an immense amount of thought and still do. My identity now also includes personal experience, thanks to working in and living through some extreme circumstances with little or no support or supervision (by this I refer to the war and post-war situations and working in a neoliberally governed academic department in the past, not madness alone). I am much more of a double agent than a wounded healer. I cannot claim that I survived anything – I knew way too much about the mental health system and didn't change enough to help myself from within. I gripped way too tight to any remaining sanity that I had, while drawing on everything I know works to help me get better. Some professionals do help. Talking does help – and for more than the six to 12 sessions currently offered by some remaining welfare states.

While those experiences don't shape all I am, they are all part of my daily life, along with many others – my ethnicity, age, gender, race, class, sexuality, the lot. Identity counts, but it is complex and multifaceted. No ally is an ally alone, just as anyone who is mad is much more than just their madness. It's whether we bother to find out. To date, counterpartal role inquiry (Heron, 1996) is the only form of knowledge generation that has really helped co-researchers and co-activists achieve the co-creation of knowledge. I'm one of those people who think that any reality is much better co-created, even if, for some of the time, some of the people in it may have slightly different or altered perceptions of it. I believe that different ways of expressing and being are the best things we can ever experience (even if, hand on heart, they can be full-on, challenging, and even scary at times).

But, even more so, I think I'm of that generation who watched one episode of *Star Trek* too many. It led to what nowadays seems to be a naive belief that we all want to live in diverse communities where we learn about each other respectfully, fight injustice and support each other in whatever we are doing, whoever we are. This is not about dependence; it's simply very fluid interdependence as we get on with our lives and try to support each other day to day. We have to carry each other; life throws too many challenges at us not to – from war and loss to poverty, just to name a few.

Today, in the second month of 2015, much of the media and even the people around me tell me and show me that we live in a time where inequalities are growing, public investment is falling and the need for support is seen as a sign of personal failure that the person concerned, alone, is responsible for remedying, and that 'success', 'impact' and 'effectiveness' are the only things worth celebrating. I am also of the generation who didn't like it that many of the professionals working in public and other services couldn't explain what they did and why they did it, and could provide little or no account of why they routinely applied particular practices. I have no time for medical protocols and interpretations of madness either. Yet I know that some of it, including medication, helps some people. The pendulum, however, shifts too much from one end of the spectrum to another. Madness doesn't submit readily to a business model, and nor should it.

What are we doing?

We have forgotten to pay heed to the bigger picture. In England, many social workers are leaving the profession three to five years after they enter it. Politicians like to blame the training social workers receive. Yet what we find out from social workers themselves is that the work is not what they expected; it's not why they got involved in the first place.

Nowadays, I mainly spend my days supporting others to learn how to become social workers. Some of the stories they tell horrify me, just as much as they horrify them. These are not stories of daily direct abuse, but they are equally enraging and abusive, at least to me. We have developed, yet again, a blind spot for such instances of silent abuse. The support people receive, particularly as funding for it is cut, equates to a persistent 'horticulturalism' in care (Barnes, 1990). Stripped of their life stories, with no one asking about, paying attention to or learning what matters to them, how they came to be labelled 'chronically mentally ill', making a proper record of it and co-acting to remedy it, people are left isolated, socially marginalised, with nothing to occupy them, with just the occasional watering and short trips into hospital when their communities have had enough of them. Even those beds are fewer and fewer; current campaigns against cuts call solely for more beds.

We aren't asking the right questions. What is the purpose of support offered? What is it trying to achieve? This bigger picture is absent. If it is to be 'support' as opposed to 'control and containment', why are we not trying to learn more about the person and what they want? Most mainstream services simply try to keep people alive/prevent suicide, contain odd behaviour in the community or, at best, work towards the co-opted recovery targets of education and employment. What if that is not what the individual concerned wants? Most of the services offered don't reflect the life story or wants of the people they are supposed to support.

We should be looking to the bigger picture and asking the bigger questions. What kind of a world do we want to live in? What do we see as fair and want for ourselves, our neighbours, our children, our families? These may seem theoretical questions, far removed from reality, yet they are becoming more and more relevant every day as inequalities and cuts in public services grow. These are the questions that drove me to live and work the way I did. No one told me to do it. No one even paid me to do it. I just made it my business to learn and do things differently as it was the only thing that made sense. If we don't take the space and time to think through the bigger picture, to shape it with others, how we live now will just make even more people even more mad, one way or another.

The fight for mad practice, policy and studies (LeFrançois, Menzies & Reaume, 2013) needs this bigger picture, beyond its own identity. It also needs allies. It needs time and for more people to find out if they can make a difference to their own and other people's lives. I think I see the revolution much more clearly now than I did at that rave in a field in England, nearly two decades ago.

References

Barnes C (1990*). 'Cabbage Syndrome': the social construction of dependence.* Basingstoke: Falmer Press.

Cutler P, Hayward R (2005). *Exploring the Usefulness of the Policy as Process Model to Mental Health NGOs Working in Eastern Europe and Central Asia.* Centre for Reflection on Mental Health Policy Research Paper. Canterbury: Interaction Press.

Heron J (1996). *Co-operative Inquiry: research into the human condition.* London: Sage.

LeFrançois BA, Menzies R, Reaume G (eds) (2013). *Mad Matters: a critical reader in Canadian mad studies.* Toronto: Canadian Scholars' Press.

THE SEARCH GOES ON

24

The search goes on

The many chapters in this book explore several possible avenues for fostering very different social responses to madness and distress. Besides clearly demonstrating the potential of first-person knowledges in such processes, they also describe the many barriers and related difficulties. Reading through the different contributions made us realise how much there is to think about, to test out and to explore. Summing up or making any concluding remarks that would close this book didn't seem appropriate. As the ones privileged to accompany the birth of these texts, we thought that ending with questions would be more valuable than trying to identify answers from what the authors are saying.

We therefore invited all the contributors to suggest questions that they think are the most important for our collective future. The questions that follow are asked without any expectations of right and wrong answers. To us, they convey a sense of hope, but also at times a hopelessness and despair that we can ever halt the sweeping tide of biomedical psychiatry.

In their thinking about how to challenge and overcome psychiatry and connect with one another in new ways, the authors are concerned with how we can resist the co-optation of our knowledge, responses and alternatives; work in genuine partnerships where power and privilege are recognised and addressed; create research opportunities that safeguard survivor values and challenge psychiatric orthodoxies; confront whiteness within and outside psychiatry; develop structures and opportunities that enable genuine alliances; hold one another's pain and support one another; facilitate changes in academia that enable survivors to work in meaningful and democratic ways, and connect our knowledges and advance Mad Studies.

We do not suggest answers to these questions. Instead, we are directing them equally to ourselves and to anybody who is determined to keep searching for a rose garden.

*   *   *

What would a rational, empathic alien with a sense of social justice make of our responses to people with mental distress? Why do we tolerate the fact that the investment in mental health services of hundreds of billion dollars worldwide produces such poor personal, social and health outcomes in people who use services? What would happen to the compulsory treatment regimes in mental health if people who use mental health services were treated on an equal basis with other citizens? What will it take for psychiatry to acknowledge and stop iatrogenic harm? What will it take for psychiatry and communities to understand that their stigmatising and skewed obsession with risk management is the 21st century equivalent to the high walls of the Victorian asylums?
Mary O'Hagan

Psychiatric diagnosis has long been the dominant frame for explaining distress and human suffering. Its rigid, though subjective, certainty ignores the complex, profound and often tragic ways that we exist in relationship to self, others and the world. Out of our connection to the world comes that most human of our capabilities: meaning making. What would be different if we came to our relationships with each other out of a sense of curiosity rather than certainty? If we saw each other as people with many stories – rather than people with many symptoms? How does an emphasis on learning from each other revolutionise the way we think about being with each other in distress?
Beth Filson

How can those of us committed to truly challenging psychiatry and developing a liberatory response to madness and distress do this in inclusive, equal and participatory ways? Taking forward Mad Studies, we will face threats from individuals and institutions who will want to silence us and subvert our efforts. We know that there are others who want to piggyback on our struggles for their own personal purposes. How do we resist such efforts to undermine or co-opt us and our struggles, while still working in democratic, humanistic and kind ways together? That for me is the key question we face and must address.
Peter Beresford

I am left with two major questions. First, is it possible for psychiatric survivors to work within mainstream mental health organisations in peer support roles (or other roles) without being co-opted? Second, is it possible for psychiatric survivors to collaborate with mental health professionals, researchers and administrators on projects of mutual interest while maintaining their integrity and being accepted as full partners? I have been grappling with these questions in my work for more than 25 years, and the jury is still out.

Darby Penney

Ultimately I wonder, is it possible to work with allies and not lose our own identities? How do users and survivors of psychiatry maintain the authority to speak for ourselves? We need to be able to engage in difficult and often controversial conversations about the roles power and privilege play in shaping definitions of 'authority', 'knowledge' and 'evidence'. This issue of ownership extends beyond the field of research and ultimately goes to the very heart of survival and the politics of identity. From the margins, how do we resist the re-appropriation of our voices, experiences and lives? What happens when others simply claim to 'be' us? How do we preserve our legacy for the future if we can no longer find ourselves in it?

Laura Prescott

Accepted norms around who gets to study whom mean that it is psychiatrists and academics who typically get to (mis)interpret and (mis)represent survivor experiences. How can we subvert these norms so that survivors are seen as legitimate owners, researchers and scholars of our individual and collective knowledge and experiences? And, because of these accepted norms, current systems for funding research are biased in favour of mainstream treatments and approaches. This means that mainstream researchers can add new therapies or services to existing services and then explore the differences between the new therapy or service and 'treatment as usual' – a self-perpetuating system. Given this, how can survivors generate funding for meaningful and in-depth transformative research?

Angela Sweeney

How do we unlearn fear of madness and stop fighting it? How do we learn acceptance of our own and other people's altered states of mind? How do we support each other through difficult times of all kinds, including those extremely difficult times, and keep nourishing the potential for change and growth that is there in each of us? Can the powerful ways in which we connect sum up

and ultimately defeat something as big and potent as psychiatry? How can our accumulated knowledge stand strong against biomedical constructs? Will psychiatry ever stop? Is stopping it at the multitude of personal and interpersonal micro levels a way to stop it globally?
Jasna Russo

Seeing how race and racism operate as a drama, my role has been to analyse the scripts and roles given to white professionals to make me a mental illness. I am privileged to be in this ongoing play; it has empowered me to provide a mirror to what white professionals have become a victim to – the unconscious ways they fear having to diagnose black men. The remaining question is – how do we challenge the perceptions we do not want to talk about? How do we expose and challenge whiteness that has become the ghost of past theories that continues to fill the context of mental health settings? I am repaired to see the damage to my soul and ask whether the possibility of writing might be the best form of reflective therapy.
Colin King

If it were impossible to correct the mental illness system, and impossible to prevent alternatives being co-opted into that system, what might remain? Assuming psych corrections are a Western institution within broader social forces, what could provide safety from the asylum? How could a non-interventionist social movement avoid corrective impositions, only to become a mentalist institution? What has already been tried, failed, improved?
Erick Fabris

Given our insatiable need to measure success, how can we create research paradigms that actually fit with our values? It seems to me that there are qualitative methods that would fit but the process is so obtuse and so too, usually, is the writing, so most people never read it.
Shery Mead

Women's alcohol problems appear to be gendered social issues requiring unconditional positive regard from committed women who, wherever possible, have survived similar situations themselves. Can such needs be accommodated in traditional 'treatment services'? How can self-worth be increased and maintained? Could an answer lie in a new style of women's centres where survivor specialists in the fields that have been shown to lie behind drinking problems, such as domestic abuse, poverty and depression, might meet women in privacy and safety? How do we circumvent a drift into medicalising what is essentially a social problem arising from inequality and a neglect of emotional needs?

Patsy Staddon

There are people with different sorts of educational backgrounds whose work is primarily informed by their own personal experiences. We are not at home in the academic world and nor do we identify with professions assigned to help us. While our experiential backgrounds don't serve as any kind of norm, they are what motivates our work and they are central to the concepts we develop. I ask myself, what kind of structures would enable us to connect, learn from each other, empower ourselves, and question and advance our work, in whichever field we do it?

Zofia Rubinsztajn

Imagine you approached a friend, an elder, a health professional, a family member or work colleague and told them that you were in pain – extreme pain from a lot of hurt – but that you didn't know why because society didn't teach you that we are hurt by the way we are treated as babies, children and teenagers, at work, in the family and in society, and by the many oppressions inflicted on us like racism, abuse, sexism, homophobia, classism, bullying, political/religious doctrines, and many more that aren't listened to. Putting all this into context and hearing the gentle words, 'There's absolutely nothing wrong with you and you are a good person', how would you feel then? How would you feel knowing you won't be medicated, labeled or diagnosed if you were to cry, scream, shake, laugh out loud, or want someone to hold you through the pain? How would you feel in a world that could hold the hurt?

Renuka Bhakta

Given the widespread tendency to prescribe psychiatric drugs, the lack of support for people to stop taking them, and the reluctance of mainstream services to research the harm these drugs can do, how do we form alliances and build expertise and knowledge in this controversial area?

Terry Simpson

Following from what I wrote in my chapter, my questions are: what stories/experiences do we miss because it is too painful/shameful in the mind of the

teller? And can there be authentic co-production if there are those who view our stories as sickness?
Dolly Sen

What needs to change in academia to enable participatory ways of working to live up to its ideals? What does it mean to build affinity while simultaneously acknowledging and working with difference? Can I find or create the radical spaces within academia that I am looking for? Spaces in which to co-research with survivors, where unnecessary asymmetries in position and privilege are not only acknowledged but are also actively challenged and reversed?
Anna Sexton

For me, the biggest question remains: how do we teach the next generation about mad people's history? What kinds of practices do we adopt to make post-secondary learning accessible and end the systemic exclusion of mad people? How do we honour and assert mad knowledge and share and apply it in order to challenge sanist ideology? How can we engage students in mad matters, teach them to think critically so that they can cut through the rhetoric and question their own complicity in systems of oppression? In posing these questions I wonder what enrages us enough to make change? What sparks lead us to dream up and build sustainable alternatives – ones that allow us to be with and support one another in times of distress?
Danielle Landry

How do we enable the new generation of Mad scholars to find a 'place' in the corporatising university: a place for teaching and mentoring students; for activist research formed within an alternative paradigm; for service that transforms university practices of 'accessibility'; for political action with/in the community? By 'place' I mean tenure track jobs with all the benefits. In Disability Studies at Ryerson we are engaged on many fronts in the real material struggle for the organisational base and cultural interpretations that will make these goals a possibility. I think about it and work on it every day. The only question is how to keep (each other) going.
Kathryn Church

Peer specialists were intended to be alternatives to the mental health system. Over time, the integration of peer specialists validated people's experiences as ex-patients, educated staff and changed the lives of their fellow peers. Some mental health providers found this difficult. As a result, co-optation became the

only way to preserve the status quo of the mental health system. Employment is an important part of recovery. So my question is, for those who choose to work in the system, can we create independent peer specialist organisations that can fight for human rights, living wages and meaningful work?
Celia Brown

What I am left with is the question whether it actually makes sense for survivors and mental health professionals to work together towards changing the mental health system? 'The system' as it is cannot be changed radically enough to avert trauma and provide meaningful and effective alternatives to those seeking support in difficult times. 'Alternatives' that arise on the fringes of the system tend to be usurped by the dominant psychiatric powers and turned into window dressing for a fundamentally misguided paradigm. Standing together before the gates of institutional psychiatry and averting anyone from entering there may be the most important endeavour in which we should be joining forces.
Peter Stastny

I am left wondering how we are to find the power to challenge the paradigm at the core of most mental health research. By paradigm, I mean the biomedical model of mental distress that continues to dominate the majority of mental health research, treatments and services carried out in the West. Until we can do this more convincingly, it will be hard for us to claim our share of the research world and make the changes to services that we want to see.
Alison Faulkner

I remain both intrigued by and mistrustful of the desire for relations in psychiatry to be described as 'partnerships', whether at 'collegial' or 'individual treatment' levels. If we were to put aside the concept of 'partnership' as either a process or goal of our work, would we lose ground or would it be liberating, and if so in what ways? What would it take for consumers/survivors to be positioned routinely as thinkers, knowers and leaders necessary to the development of quality work, and what changes would we then start to see? What material and intellectual conditions would foster the ongoing development of our conceptual work – our unique 'discipline'– and what might the role of our allies be in all of this?
Cath Roper

Many people who age with madness are isolated and either grow silent or difficult to understand for people who don't know them. Professional, bureaucratised,

risk-assessing accounts of their lives take over. How can we ensure their voices, worlds and stories remain listened to and interacted with, free of isolation and professional dominance over their lives?
Reima Ana Maglajlic

Contributors

Peter Beresford OBE is Emeritus Professor of Social Policy at Brunel University London and Professor of Citizen Participation at the University of Essex. He is a long term user/survivor of mental health services and Co-Chair of Shaping Our Lives, the independent UK disabled people's and service users' organisation and network (http://www.shapingourlives.org.uk/). He has a longstanding interest in issues of participation as a researcher, writer, campaigner, educator and service user, and a longstanding interest in personalisation and person-centred support. He is author of *A Straight Talking Guide to Being a Mental Health Service User* (PCCS Books, 2010) and his latest book is *All Our Welfare: towards participatory social policy* (Policy Press, 2016).

Renuka Bhakta qualified as a social worker in 1992 and for the next eight years worked in a variety of related jobs while also coping with depression. Her hospitalisation in the psychiatric system in 2000 led to her strong commitment to the user movement and survivor-led models of mental health work. She worked with organisations such as Lambeth Mind, Southwark Mind, Mental Fight Club, CoolTan Arts and the Save Lives, Save Amardeep Campaign, which won the Sheila McKechnie Foundation London Social Justice Award 2009. She has also worked with South London & Maudsley NHS Trust and the Mental Health Foundation in developing training and research. Renuka set up Alternatives in Mental Health and Kindred Minds, both projects that promote creative ways to wellbeing. Renuka is also a key leader in mental health liberation work within the UK Re-evaluation

Counselling communities and an engaged Buddhist and facilitator of mindfulness. Her vision is to promote the art of living well without the use of psychiatric drugs and she currently works at a London GP practice as a wellbeing adviser.

Celia Brown is a psychiatric survivor who was instrumental in developing the first peer specialist civil service title in the US. A long-time activist and leader in the psychiatric survivor movement, she is a former board member of the National Association for Rights Protection and Advocacy (NARPA), and was a founding member of the National People of Color Consumer/Survivor Network. Celia is Board President of MindFreedom International and serves as the organisation's primary representative to the United Nations on the International Convention for Human Rights for People with Disabilities. Celia is the Regional Advocacy Specialist at the New York State Office of Mental Health. She trains and advises people with psychosocial disabilities and their families. She is a field school graduate of the Center to Study Recovery in Social Contexts, Nathan Klein Institute. Celia has presented nationally and internationally on topics such as self-help, peer counselling, advocacy, trauma and cultural competency.

Kathryn Church is Director of the School of Disability Studies at Ryerson University in Toronto. For more than a decade she has been part of key initiatives that have brought the programme's 'vision, passion, action' message to life across the university and in the public eye. Kathryn is a mad-positive academic engaged in the activist project of blending disability and Mad studies. Her involvement as a Mad movement ally dates back 30 years to the first articulations of 'consumer participation' and the use of psychiatric survivor narratives in/against mental health policy formation. Author of *Forbidden Narratives: critical autobiography as social science* (Routledge, 1996) and co-editor of *Learning through Community* (Springer, 2008), she wrote a dozen documents for psychiatric survivor-led organisations doing local economic development, and was consultant to and did international circulation for the documentary film *Working Like Crazy* (National Film Board of Canada, 1999). Kathryn is an award-winning instructor and curator of research-based exhibitions. In 2015 she received a Woman of Distinction award from the Ontario Confederation of University Faculty Associations, and a David C. Onley Award for Leadership in Accessibility.

Bhargavi Davar PhD is a childhood survivor of psychiatric institutions in India and has survived psychosocial disability through use of non-medical approaches. She has worked extensively in the field of mental health research and advocacy since 1993. She worked independently as a social science researcher, writing and publishing on gender, culture and mental health. She has published several books, including *Psychoanalysis as a Human Science* (Sage, 1995), *Mental Health of Indian Women* (Sage, 1999), *Mental Health from a Gender Perspective* (Sage, 2001) and *Gendering Mental Health: knowledges, identities, institutions* (Oxford University Press, 2015). She founded the Bapu Trust for Research on Mind and Discourse in 1999, to give an organisational framework to her human rights work. Bhargavi is a trained arts-based therapist, devotes herself to giving support to families and users who experience 'extreme states' and is the director of a community-based mental health programme in Pune slums, where she lives.

Erick Fabris was one of the 'West End Psychiatric Survivors' who started Psychiatric Survivor Pride Day in Toronto in the 1990s. His work with Pride, and later the No Force Coalition and several other actions, led him to look into Community Treatment Orders for his MA thesis. He published a book on this topic in 2011, titled *Tranquil Prisons* (University of Toronto Press). Erick currently works on mad cultural events in Toronto.

Alison Faulkner is a survivor researcher and trainer in mental health with an interest in the role and value of experiential knowledge and personal narratives. She has over 25 years' experience of mental health research and consultancy, including working for the Mental Health Foundation, NSUN (the National Survivor User Network), Mind, Together and the Joseph Rowntree Foundation. Alison's own experience of using mental health services includes inpatient care, medication, psychotherapy and crisis services. She has written and presented extensively on the subject from a user/survivor perspective. She is currently working with NSUN on national standards for involvement and is studying for her PhD at City University, London.

Beth Filson is a writer, educator, and self-taught artist. She has been involved with the development of the internationally renowned curriculum in Intentional Peer Support and peer support alternatives to the psychiatric system. Her experience with multiple hospitalisations early on informs the work she does today in integrating trauma understanding and approaches in both primary care settings and the mental health system. Currently she is involved in the development of proactive planning interventions to eliminate seclusion and restraint in inpatient psych settings and reduce the conditions that lead to severe distress and coercive practices. Beth has worked with diverse groups including mental health organisations, the criminal justice system and communities devastated by both natural and man-made disasters. She co-authored the manual *Engaging Women in Trauma-Informed Peer Support: a guide* (2012) for the National Center for Trauma-Informed Care and Alternatives to Seclusion and Restraint. Her art has been exhibited widely in the southeastern region of the US. Beth is also an award-winning poet. She lives in Western Massachusetts.

Maths Jesperson was born in 1954. Since 1988 he has worked as a regional officer of the Swedish National Organization for Social and Mental Health (RSMH). He was a founding member of the European Network of (ex-) Users and Survivors of Psychiatry (ENUSP) in 1991, and is still active in the network. Maths was the initiator, the leader and later a board member of PO-Skåne, a professional service that provides personal ombudsmen for people with severe psychosocial disabilities. In January 2006 he presented PO-Skåne at a seminar in the United Nations headquarters in New York as an example of supported decision-making. The seminar was connected to the UN committee working on the UN Convention on the Rights of Persons with Disabilities. Since then he has presented PO-Skåne in Oslo, Copenhagen, Dublin, Killarney, Brussels, Trier, Alzey, Berlin, Vienna, Eisenstadt, Lisbon, Florence, Ljubljana, Belgrade, Sofia, Budapest, Prague, Riga and Santiago de Chile.

Colin King is a normal, sweet and colourless personality, coloured by the power of the diagnosis 'schizophrenia'. He travelled the escalator of madness in the corridors of English schools, the hospitality of the prison services and the civilisation of Englishness. He wishes to thank all those who nicknamed him as educationally subnormal and injected him with a free cocktail of medication. These privileges have inspired an energy to offer free counselling to those he has made visible – European psychiatry. Colin is an ex-mental health practitioner, a researcher and an enabler of whiteness who wants to be freed from drapetomania. He is still a slave and still enslaved to a system that has no time for his heritage.

Danielle Landry is a mad-identified PhD student in sociology at York University. Her research interests include accessibility in the workplace and survivor-led research. She enjoys working part time as an instructor in the School of Disability Studies at Ryerson University in Toronto. She is currently involved in the community as a member of the Psychiatric Disabilities Anti-Violence Coalition (PDAC) and as a board member for the Empowerment Council. On her days off you are likely to find her playing in the green spaces in Toronto.

Brenda A LeFrançois is a professor at Memorial University of Newfoundland. She engages in mad activist scholarship in the areas of children's agency and psychiatrisation, the lived experience of sanism, and organising alternatives to mainstream services. Brenda has published many journal articles on these topics and is co-editor of three volumes, including (along with Canadian scholars and activists Robert Menzies and Geoffrey Reaume) the book *Mad Matters: a critical reader in Canadian Mad Studies* (Canadian Scholars' Press Inc, 2013). She has been an activist for over 20 years, aiming always to bridge the divide between academia and mad communities. She is currently working with local communities to develop the Hearing Voices Network for Atlantic Canada. Brenda has two lovely daughters, a loving partner, and several cats.

Reima Ana Maglajlic is a senior lecturer in social work at the University of Sussex in England. Originally from Croatia, she first worked briefly as a social worker for refugees and displaced persons in her home town of Zagreb, before moving in 1994 to learn more about social work from Professor David Brandon at Anglia Ruskin University in Cambridge. She later worked with Professor Brandon at Shield, a practice and research centre based at the university that supported practice development and research on alternatives to mainstream health and social care. Everything important that she knows about mental health, she learned from him. In 1999 she moved to Sarajevo, Bosnia and Herzegovina, initially as a project manager for a TEMPUS-funded project to establish an MA in Community Mental Health at the Universities of Banja Luka and Sarajevo. Subsequently, she moved between freelance work in south-east Europe and academia in the UK. Between 2011 and 2013, she was Research and Monitoring Director at the Mental Disability Advocacy Centre in Budapest.

Shery Mead has been developing and teaching Intentional Peer Support since 1995. Intentional Peer Support is a way of thinking about and inviting transformative relationships between people. In this process we learn to use relationships to see ourselves from new angles, develop greater awareness of personal and relational patterns and support and challenge each other in trying out new ways of seeing and knowing. Shery has presented and trained extensively, nationally and internationally, on the topics of alternative approaches to crisis, trauma-informed peer services, systems change and the development and implementation of peer-operated services. Her publications include academic articles, training manuals and a book co-authored with Mary Ellen Copeland, *Wellness Recovery Action Planning and Peer Support* (Peach Press, 2004).

Mary O'Hagan was a key initiator of the mental health service user movement in New Zealand in the late 1980s and was the first chairperson of the World Network of Users and Survivors of Psychiatry between 1991 and 1995. She has been an advisor to the United Nations and the World Health Organisation. Mary was a full-time Mental Health Commissioner in New Zealand between 2000 and 2007. She has written and spoken extensively on recovery and user/survivor perspectives in many countries. Mary is now an international consultant in mental health and runs a social enterprise that has developed PeerZone – peer-led workshops in mental health and addiction. She is also leading the development of Swell, an online recovery toolkit for people with mental distress and the people who work with them. Mary has published a memoir, *Madness Made Me*.

Darby Penney MLS is a long-time activist in the human rights movement for people with psychiatric histories and President of the Community Consortium, a peer-run, non-profit organisation working for the social inclusion of people with psychiatric labels. She is a co-author of *Engaging Women in Trauma-Informed Peer Support: a guidebook* (National Center for Trauma-Informed Care, 2012) and, with Cathy Cave, has developed curricula and delivered trauma-informed peer support training to hundreds of people across the US. Darby was previously Director of Recipient Affairs at the New York State Office of Mental Health, where she brought the perspectives of people with psychiatric histories into the policymaking process. She is co-author with Peter Stastny of *The Lives They Left Behind: suitcases from a state hospital attic* (Bellevue Literary Press, 2008), based on a study of the lives of state hospital inmates from the 19th and 20th centuries, and a website, www.suitcaseexhibit.org. She is Principal Investigator in a new study examining the effectiveness of Intentional Peer Support (IPS) in improving community living and participation for adults with psychiatric disabilities.

Laura Prescott is a long-time human rights activist, feminist, research and policy consultant and artist living near Sedona, Arizona. She founded Sister Witness International Inc, in order to address the violence permeating the lives of women and girls who have been psychiatrically institutionalised. For over 20 years she has worked for federal, state and international governmental and non-governmental agencies. Her primary concentration has been eliminating coercive practices and creating gender-specific, trauma-informed approaches for women and girls who have survived atrocity. Laura recently became a certified Holotropic Breathwork™ facilitator and is excited about the possibilities of this non-medical alternative. She has presented in over 36 states in the US and 10 countries throughout

Europe, the Middle East, Latin America and Asia, and has published widely on a variety of topics. She is a survivor of violence and a psychiatric ex-patient and can be reached at www.sisterwitnessinternational.org or lpswi@aol.com

Cath Roper has a BA, a DipEd and a Masters in Social Health. She held one of four pioneering staff-consumer consultant positions in mental health services in Victoria between 1995 and 1999 and later became the first person to occupy a consumer academic role in Australia, at the Centre for Psychiatric Nursing, University of Melbourne. Cath experienced annual involuntary admissions to mental health services over a 13-year period. She has a strong interest in working alongside clinicians towards practices that support the self-determination of people subject to mental health legislation and reduce restrictive practices in mental health services. She delivers education and training in academic and specialist mental health service settings across Victoria, including co-ordinating a mandatory consumer perspective subject as part of the Postgraduate Diploma in Nursing, Mental Health at the University of Melbourne. Cath is well known for her dedication to promoting consumer leadership and co-production.

Zofia Rubinsztajn has worked for the last 10 years in a Berlin-based, survivor-controlled project for women and trans people who experienced sexual violence as children. Prior to that she worked for several years at a rape hot line and in an autonomous shelter for battered women and children. And prior to all that she travelled through different worlds. Besides the obvious focus on (sexual) violence, Zofia's work centres on related themes that also connect to her experiential background. These include drug use, sex work, suicidality, voice-hearing and self-harm.

Jasna Russo comes from the former Yugoslavia and is based in Berlin, Germany, where she works as an independent researcher. She is a long-term activist in the international user/survivor movement. Jasna has an MA in clinical psychology and has worked on both survivor-controlled and collaborative research projects, including several large-scale international studies. Her work has been published in anthologies and journals in Germany and the UK. In 2011 Jasna was the main organiser of the international conference 'Searching for a Rose Garden: fostering real alternatives to psychiatry', which inspired this book. Her main interest is in exploring the accumulated knowledge of people treated as mad or 'mentally ill' and whether we can connect across the globe to jointly develop our own first person-defined model of madness.

Dolly Sen is a writer, film-maker mental health consultant and trainer, with lived experience of psychosis, mood disorder and PTSD. Her training and public speaking has taken her to the World Health Organisation in Geneva, Oxford University, The Barbican, the Mayor of London, the University of Westminster, Guy's Hospital, the Probation Service and over 100 charity, corporate and statutory organisations. She has written over 10 books and contributed chapters to more than 20 others, such as *The World is Full of Laughter* (Chipmunkapublishing, 2002) and *Our Encounters with Suicide* (PCCS Books, 2013). Dolly has made over 30 media appearances on TV, radio, the internet and in print. Her other mental health work involves consultancy, keynote speaking, coaching, research, group facilitation, campaigning, social media and creative work.

Anna Sexton has trained as a professional archivist and has had several roles in the archival field, including managing the archives service for the City of Peterborough. She has recently completed a PhD in the Department of Information Studies at University College London, where she is currently working as a sessional lecturer. Her PhD research explores participatory approaches to building life history archives in the context of mental health. Her PhD writing is auto-ethnographic and seeks to unravel and trace the complex threads of power, authority and control that run through participatory processes. Her PhD research speaks to the broader questions around archival endeavours approached within a social justice framework as well as offering some specific insights into archival work that seeks to document mental health from the perspective of the individual with lived experience.

Clare Shaw is a key figure in the UK self-injury survivor movement. A founding member of the STEPS self-help group for women who self-injure and the Liverpool-based radical campaigns group Mad Women, Clare has drawn from her academic background as well as her own personal experiences to inform her work and publications around issues including self-injury, sexual abuse and borderline personality disorder. This combination of personal, academic and campaigning experience also informs Clare's work as a teacher and trainer. In 2006 Clare co-founded *harm-ed*, a user-led self-injury training organisation. After leaving the organisation in 2013, Clare continues to work on a freelance, independent basis, informing services and influencing practice across the UK and beyond. She is also Royal Literary Fellow at the University of Huddersfield.

Terry Simpson was Co-ordinator of the United Kingdom Advocacy Network (UKAN), a national survivor led organisation, from 1993 to 2002. He was a founding member of Leeds Survivor Led Crisis Service, Leeds Mental Health Advocacy Group and Leeds Survivors Poetry, and is currently on the board of the Sunrise Center, an international project to help people come off psychiatric drugs. He co-edited a poetry anthology by mental health survivors, *And The World Really Had Changed* (LSP Press, 1996), a collection of short stories, *The Mind Machine* (Local Voices Publications, 2006), and a CD of writing and verse, *Soul Survivors* (2008). He also edited a collection of stories about recovery from mental health problems, *Doorways in the Night* (Local Voices, 2004). Two of his play scripts about the mental health system have been filmed for use on Open University courses and he won the 2001 Martha Robinson Poetry Competition and the 2010 Notre Voix/Our Voice international poetry competition.

Patsy Staddon recovered from two decades of problem drinking in 1988. She returned to university, gaining her PhD in the sociology of women's alcohol use and its treatment in 2009. She is particularly interested in theorising the politics of women's drinking and in developing holistic and non-judgemental responses, within the context of small, women-only groups and a supportive helpline that is well networked with specialists in the field of domestic abuse, self-harm and depression. She has a keen interest in mental health as a whole and is very active in the field. In 2013 she edited *Mental Health Service Users in Research: a critical sociological perspective* (Policy Press) and is involved a good deal locally as a service user and a carer, as well as a practising (retired!) academic and chair of the organisation she founded, Women's Independent Alcohol Support (WIAS). Her edited book, *Women and Alcohol: social perspectives* (Policy Press), was published in June 2015.

Peter Stastny is a New York-based psychiatrist, documentary film-maker and a co-founder of the International Network Toward Alternatives and Recovery. He is a lecturer at the Global Mental Health Program of Columbia University and until recently was a consultant to the New York City Department of Mental Health in connection with the New York City Parachute Project. This federally-funded project aims to redesign crisis responses for individuals experiencing acute psychosis and altered states that interfere with their independence and community life. Peter has frequently collaborated with psychiatric survivors by spearheading peer specialist services and peer-run businesses, as well as in research and writing projects. Examples are a book (with Darby Penney) called

The Lives They Left Behind: suitcases from a state hospital attic (Bellevue Literary Press, 2008) and the edited volume *Alternatives Beyond Psychiatry*, with Peter Lehmann (Peter Lehman Publishing, 2007). Peter has directed a number of documentary and experimental films, many dealing with the experiences of survival and recovery.

Angela Sweeney was part of her local survivor movement as a teenager and young adult and conducted her first survivor research project as an undergraduate student in 1998. Sometime after graduating she joined the Sainsbury Centre for Mental Health to work with Jan Wallcraft on a study of the British Survivor Movement, *On Our Own Terms* (Sainsbury Centre for Mental Health, 2003), before moving to the Service User Research Enterprise (SURE) at the Institute of Psychiatry, where she gained a PhD in medical sociology. She has a particular interest in survivor-controlled research, trauma-informed approaches, survivors' perspectives on and experiences of psychiatric services and treatments, and alternatives to mainstream biomedical psychiatry, including trauma and social models of causation. She is currently undertaking a five-year post-doctoral fellowship exploring assessment processes for talking therapies, and divides her time between this and looking after her two spirited young daughters.

David Webb completed what is thought to be the world's first PhD on suicide by a survivor in 2006, followed in 2010 by his book *Thinking about Suicide* (PCCS Books). After many years as a (psychosocial) disability advocate/activist, chronic illness has forced him into early retirement and he now lives quietly in Castlemaine (Australia), an old gold rush town near Melbourne.

INDEX